NOM
YOURSELF

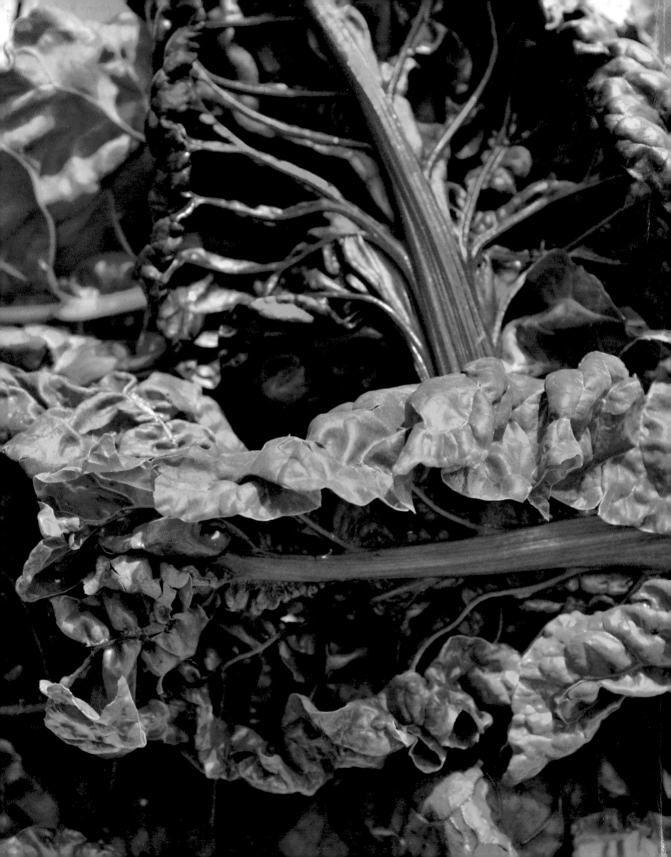

NOM YOURSELF

Simple Vegan Cooking

MARY MATTERN

AVERY
an imprint of Penguin Random House
New York

AVERY

an imprint of Penguin Random House LLC
375 Hudson Street
New York, New York 10014

Most Avery books are available at special quantity discounts for bulk purchase
for sales promotions, premiums, fund-raising, and educational needs. Special books
or book excerpts also can be created to fit specific needs. For details,
write SpecialMarkets@penguinrandomhouse.com.

ISBN: 978-1-58333-585-7

Printed in the United States of America
1   3   5   7   9   10   8   6   4   2

BOOK DESIGN BY SHUBHANI SARKAR

Neither the publisher nor the author is engaged in rendering professional advice
or services to the individual reader. The ideas, procedures, and suggestions contained
in this book are not intended as a substitute for consulting with your physician. All
matters regarding your health require medical supervision. Neither the author nor the
publisher shall be liable or responsible for any loss or damage allegedly
arising from any information or suggestion in this book.

The recipes contained in this book have been created for the ingredients and
techniques indicated. The publisher is not responsible for your specific health or
allergy needs that may require supervision. Nor is the publisher responsible for any
adverse reactions you may have to the recipes contained in the book, whether you follow
them as written or modify them to suit your personal dietary needs or tastes.

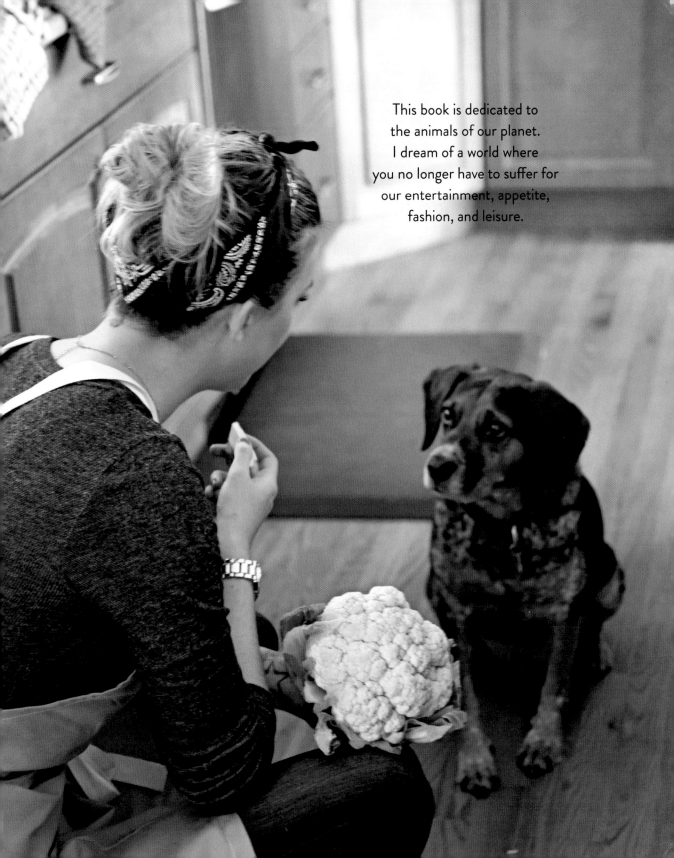

This book is dedicated to
the animals of our planet.
I dream of a world where
you no longer have to suffer for
our entertainment, appetite,
fashion, and leisure.

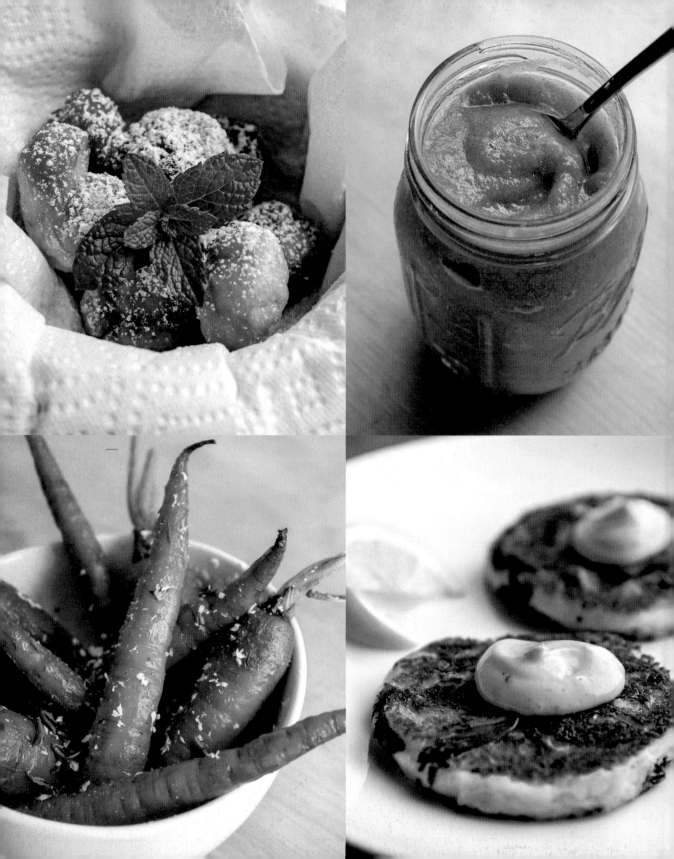

CONTENTS

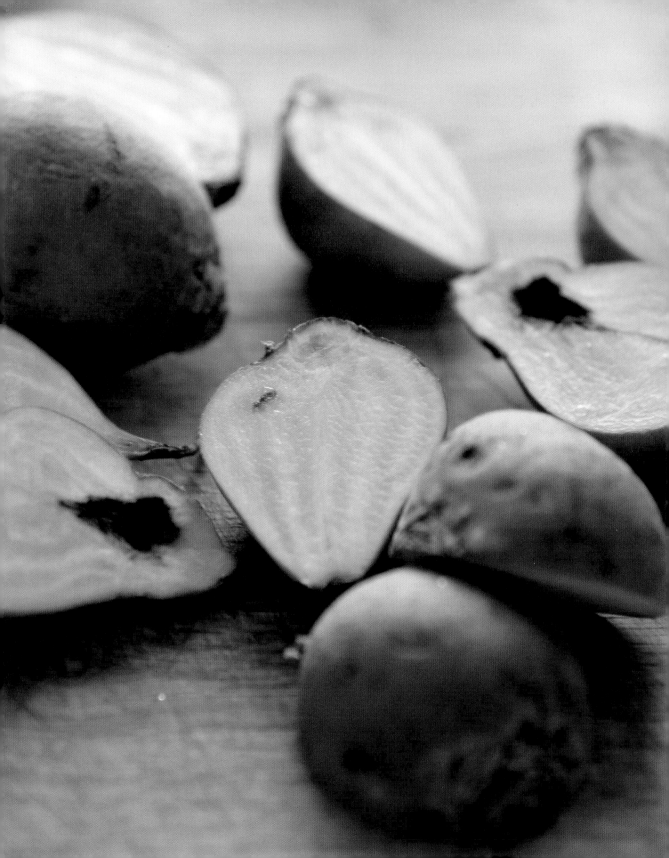

FOREWORD

> The two most
> important days in
> your life are the day
> you are born and the
> day you find out why.
>
> **—MARK TWAIN**

THE QUOTE REALLY SUMS IT UP. WHEN THE FUEL OF passion drives us, and that passion comes from a place of wanting to leave an impact and make a difference, there is nothing that will get in our way. Social media, as we all know, has become the greatest microphone we have to reach the masses and share our personal story and our purpose, and it can inspire others within this virtual community. From the beginning of time, food has brought people together, and it is our innate instinct to share meals with others within our community. Through the power of virtual platforms we are able to build on this surreal sense of community by sharing the foods and moments in time that inspire us daily.

I was first introduced to the power of plants at a young age and was determined to scream it from the mountaintops to whoever would listen. Being an activist at heart, I learned quickly that our forks are the greatest tools we have to make a difference for the animals, our health, and the planet.

Eating vegan has grown far beyond a trend, and just in the past few years it seems to have become a key piece of the conversation within the culinary world. More and more chefs are starting to recognize that showcasing plants is not only a healthier option but a channel of innovation and creativity that is gaining momentum. We are at the brink of a very exciting time, and we all need to do our part to support this snowballing movement.

Mary Mattern is a perfect example of someone who has taken her love for food, passion for cooking, and compassion for animals as an opportunity to build an online community to share just how easy it is to eat and embrace a vegan diet with simple, plant-based, comforting foods. I cannot tell you how many times I have seen a Nom Yourself post on social media and started craving some vegan comfort food. Mary is a mover and a shaker; she brings others together with the foods she posts, keeping us all hungry and constantly inspiring folks to get back in the kitchen. With the foods that strike that memory or emotional connection we have from childhood, the comfort foods we love is where Mary's food shines. Her work has reached people around the world, and she inspires us all daily with the message not only that vegan cooking is approachable and delicious, but also that when we embrace our personal passion, our purpose for making a difference, there is no stopping us and we can create the path we desire.

It is so amazing to see the culinary journey unfolding for Mary and to know that her creative work is getting the recognition it deserves. This book is a wonderful showcase of that work. We are very lucky to have such a passionate influencer in the vegan community who is truly living her purpose and supporting others to do the same, starting in the kitchen.

CHAD SARNO
Chef, educator, and plant-pusher
www.chadsarno.com
www.rouxbe.com/plant-based

ACKNOWLEDGMENTS

I'VE BEEN SO VERY LUCKY TO HAVE THE GREATEST support system by my side during the cooking and writing process of this book. I would not have been able to complete *Nom Yourself* without the encouragement and love from my friends and family.

I would like to thank my parents, Richard and Kathyrn, for raising me to be a compassionate, determined, and artistic human being. You make me want to be a better person every single day. I have no words for the love and commitment you have shown me over the years. Thank you for believing in my dreams and allowing me to follow them with your full support.

I'd also like to thank my sister and brother, Elizabeth and Brian, for believing in me. You guys amaze me every day and I am so glad that you have shared this crazy journey with me, even when it may seem that you have no idea what it is I'm doing. I love you guys.

I would have never started this cooking journey without the help of an amazing kitchen in Baltimore and the roommate who came along with it. Lisa Dietrich, thanks for putting up with dirty dishes and my early-morning and late-night cooking sessions. Without that beautiful stove of yours, I would not be writing this right now.

Bryan Miranda, thank you for supporting me throughout this whole entire writing process. I will never forget the moments we shared while this book was being created. Jim, Barbara, Matt, Danielle, and Jackie, I am forever thankful to have met you. Your support and love throughout the writing of this book means a lot to me.

With this book I will continue to move forward as an activist, cook, and artist and strive to be the best human being I can be. I would not be able to do so without the continued support of the family that has so lovingly taken me in as their own. Team Fallon-Yeskey, thanks for believing in me from day one. Mary Alice, Dave, Spencer, Josh, and Dexter, there's nothing we can't fix with duct tape and construction paper.

Chad Sarno, thank you for inspiring me from the very beginning of my journey with food that has truly opened my mind to knowing that the possibilities are endless in the kitchen. Your foreword here, as well as wise words of advice throughout the past two years, have humbled me and make me fall in love with cooking all over again, every single day.

Honorable Mentions: Very special thank-yous to the Mattern family, the Benson family, the Ellsworth family (love you, Matt and Jennifer), Kathryn Pollak-Gorman, Jackie Smith, Sarah Smith, the Smith family, the Horn family, the DelleDonne family, Christine Prenez, Melissa Danis, Tom Cragg, the Austins, Andrew Gabriel, Kim Juretic, Cara Schrock, the Schrock family, Gabrielle Becker, Tony Kanal, Brendan Brazier, Kate Lewis, Lucia Watson, Gigi Campo, Marc Gerald, Lucy Wearing, Vivek Venkatraman, Augusto Pagliarini, Toby Morse, Moby, Ruth Tal, Ellie Goulding, Jamey Jasta, Aaron Elliott (BP), Steve Berra, Chris Rubenstein, Hunter Burgan, Hiram Camillo, Tommy Rasera, Corissa Jones, Anne Thornton, Kim Jones, Timothy Shieff, Kevin Minto (I got my rematch and lost), Jeremy Piven, Dan Elswick, Chris Perino, Sajin Price, The Vegan Zombie, Douglas Gautraud, Luca Enrico Fantini, Andy Coverdale, George Watsky (for the CC album that helped me write this book), Scales and Nappy Roots, Mercy For Animals, The Humane Society of the United States, the Baltimore Orioles, and Baltimore City.

Just writing this out, I've realized just how many people have truly affected my life and the process by which this book was developed. Very grateful for the knowledge and support you have given me.

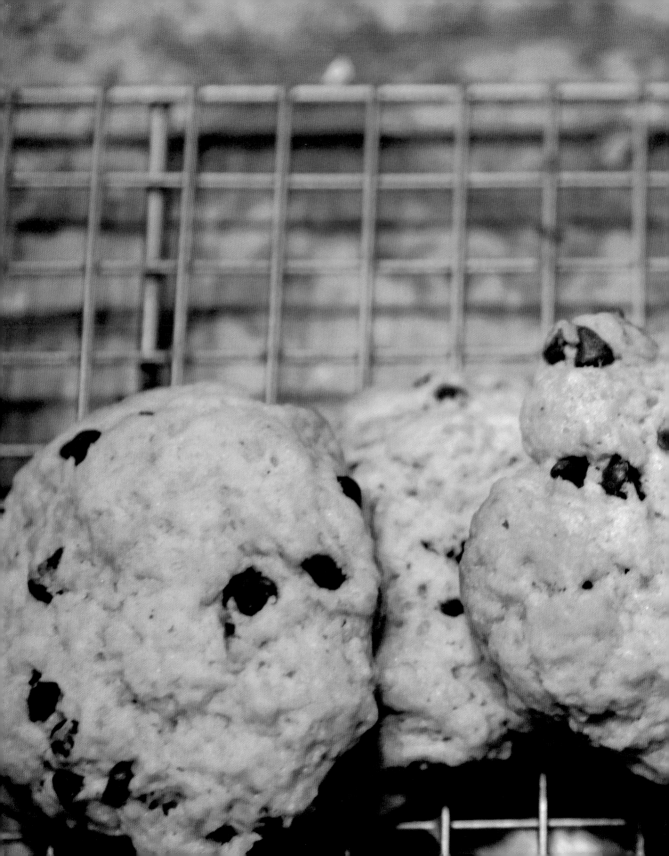

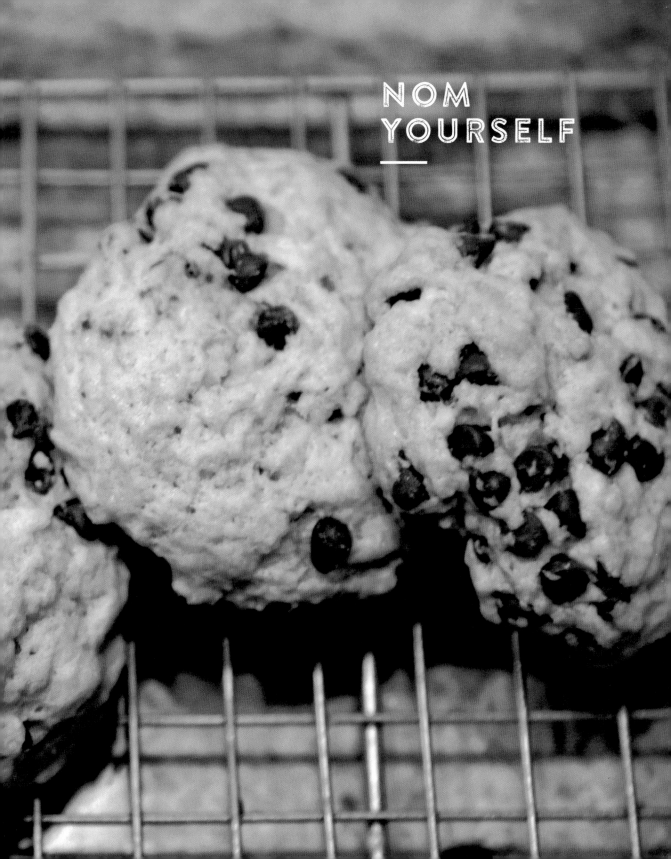

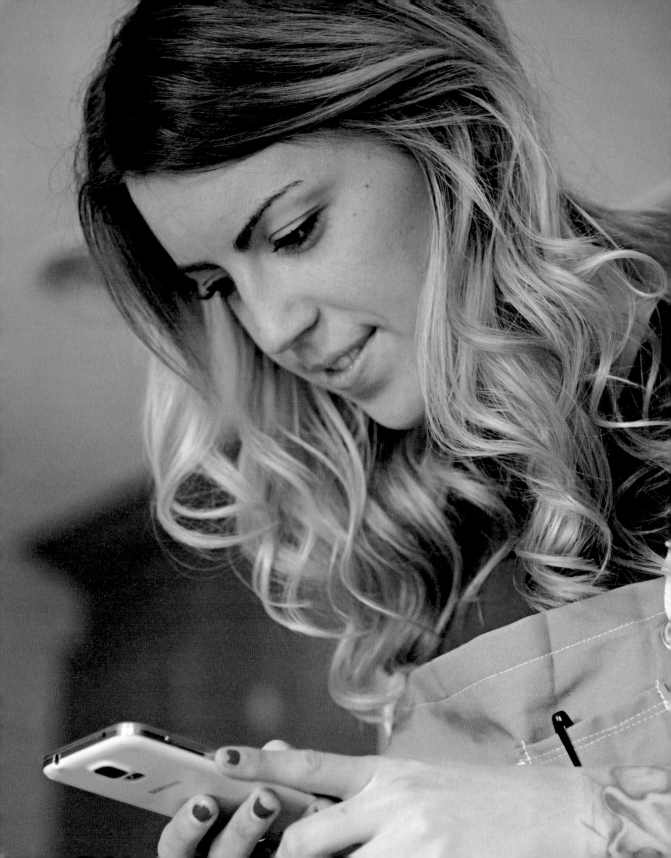

INTRODUCTION

EDWARD NORTON ONCE SAID, "INSTEAD OF TELLING the world what you're eating for breakfast, you can use social networking to do something that's meaningful." Well, with all respect to Mr. Norton, I think I manage to do both on a daily basis. When I post a picture of pancakes on my Nom Yourself website or Instagram, hundreds to thousands of people view it, drool a little bit, send a screenshot to their friends, and then realize—wow, that delicious, decadent, rich dish is vegan!

Every day, through my presence online, I show people how amazingly delicious vegan food can be. And I gently suggest to the meat-and-potatoes crowd that a vegan lifestyle really doesn't mean a life of deprivation. Eating a plant-based diet actually means a fuller, happier life, one that's compassionate, healthy, and creative.

Hundreds of my followers who previously thought "I could never go vegan" or "Where would I get my protein if I cut out eggs?!" have been inspired by my photos and stories to make the commitment. And I hope this book will inspire you the same way. So I'll keep right on posting my breakfast pictures, thank you very much—and you should, too!

WHERE IT ALL BEGAN

I am who I am today because of the first two people I met when I came into this world—my parents, Richard and Kathryn. Richard is the guy in line who will start a conversation with anyone, regardless of where he is or who you are. He taught me that we must treat everyone equally and that you can learn something from everyone. Kathryn is a woman with a lot of love who gives it all to her children. She's shown me that being myself should always be my number one priority and there isn't a thing in the world that can't be fixed with a good laugh. Along with my siblings, Elizabeth and Brian, we are a family of best friends. We have stuck together through thick and thin—and there have been a lot of both.

I grew up in the suburbs of New York City, in a little town called Suffern, just far enough away from the hustle and bustle of the big city to see the stars at night but close enough to know why they call it the city that never sleeps. So naturally, I became the New York City teenager who got her first tattoo at sixteen in the basement of a shop that also sold hookahs, Bob Marley T-shirts, and those fluorescent posters that for some reason always feature frogs and mushrooms. I sprawled in Union Square on weekends and watched people shop, dance, fight, love, and live.

With its subway performers, street dancers, and never-ending concerts, New York City quickly made me fall in love with music. So at the young age of seventeen, I boldly quit high school and started traveling the country with musicians, selling their merchandise. This isn't something I recommend everyone do. I love learning and value education greatly, but I personally benefited more from being on the road. For four years I studied the music industry and learned it inside and out. I woke up each morning in a different zip code and explored the cuisine and culture of what felt like every city and town across America.

After years of the road-tripping lifestyle that came with being a merch girl, I settled into a job as a label manager in Baltimore, a city I knew nothing about (beyond having watched a few episodes of *The Wire*). After working in the music industry, I was looking for a place to call home. When I started to really dig into Baltimore, I had what I guess you could call a quarter-life crisis—but the good kind. I felt compelled to explore what I wanted out of life. I found myself asking, *Who am I? What am I all about? What do I love and value most? What changes could I make to become a better person?* After lots of introspection, I decided to spend a year finding out what Baltimore had to offer me and, even more important, what I had to offer it.

So let me take you back to my life right before Nom Yourself. To give myself more flexibility and time on my soul-searching quest, I quit the music business and became a nanny for a wonderful family of three—an incredible little boy named Spencer, his loving and strong mother, Mary Alice, and his witty father, Dave. My relationship with this family as their nanny is one that I will be forever grateful for. They took me in as part of their family, and took me to my first farmers market, a debt I can never repay. Every Saturday morning, Mary Alice and I would trek to the Waverly Farmers Market and see what gorgeous produce was for sale. I'd explore heirloom tomatoes, and Mary Alice would show me how to pick the perfect peaches. Surrounded by lush kale, fragrant strawberries, and stubbornly knobby, hearty beets, I fell completely in love with the bounty I saw on offer. But when I came home, arms loaded with arugula and parsnips, I realized one thing: I had no idea how to cook.

Right around this time, I moved to a new house in order to live with my friend Lisa. The kitchen in this house was a wonder. It was gorgeous, spacious, filled with natural light, inviting—and it had its quirks, too. It made me work to enjoy it. I had to light the oven with a match any time I wanted to use it. At first, that seemed like a pain, but once I lit it successfully by myself, it made me curious about what else I could accomplish in this kitchen. Somehow the space made me feel both at home and inspired. I wanted to make the kitchen—and myself—proud of the meals I would create here. The kitchen was telling me, "This is your chance!"

I'd like to tell you that I fell in love with cooking the first day I decided to give it a shot, but that is far from the truth. I was frustrated for a couple of weeks (though it felt like forever). I'd bring home delicious asparagus and parsnips, painstakingly chop them and coat them with olive oil—and burn them to a crisp. My muffins wouldn't rise, my eggplant ended up too soggy, and I could never wait for my avocados

to ripen enough before slicing into them. So many times I would be about to say "screw it" and order takeout, but something inside me would push back. It was something I hadn't felt before—this immense sense of creativity.

So I persisted, trying new spices and new ingredients each day. I woke up at five a.m. to get into the kitchen, and in those early-dawn hours I learned to dice, mince, sauté, and sear. I also learned to take a morning photograph with natural sunlight (which I know now is the key to taking great food photos at home). To put it simply, I fell in love with cooking.

At first I followed recipes, and as I tried more and more of them, my pantry became stocked with what I now realize are essential staples to have on hand: olive oil, flour, sea salt, and more (you can see my full list on page 5). But soon it started to feel wrong to go to the bustling market and focus only on the specific ingredients for a recipe while ignoring the other luscious-looking vegetables just because they weren't on my grocery list. So once I felt like I had a handle on how to put a dish together, I tossed the lists! I started shopping by season, picking the most vibrantly colored and delicious fruits and vegetables each time I visited the market and figuring out what to do with them once I got home.

Cooking with what was available in the kitchen and the garden was a challenge that I welcomed with open arms. Sure, sometimes I would ask myself, *What the hell is kale and why did I decide it was a good idea to buy five pounds of the stuff?* But experimenting with new ingredients always turned into a fun, fascinating journey of discovery. I also started to become much more knowledgeable about what exactly I was putting into my body.

In the kitchen, I loved to cook inventively and imagine new flavor combinations, and I loved to take photos of my results. I liked to think of my creations as edible art—art that anyone with the desire to get into the kitchen could make. What's more, I felt *great* and I wanted the world to know it. Once I realized how easy and fulfilling it was to make amazing food from the earth's bounty, I wanted to inspire others to do exactly what I was doing.

So I started posting photos on Instagram. My first followers were, of course, my friends and family. They were seeing a side of me that hadn't been present for quite some time at that point: passion. I was happily transforming into a walking, talking fountain of knowledge about cooking, gardening, farming, and produce. As they followed my posts, they soon noticed a pattern forming. Apparently I had taken meat, poultry, fish, eggs, and dairy out of my diet. I say "they noticed" because, honestly, I hadn't.

These days, people ask me all the time how I became vegan. I'm sure you vegans out there will relate, since usually the second question people ask when you tell anyone you're vegan is how it happened (the first one, obviously, is, "But how do you get your protein?"). My answer is always: I became vegan through cooking. Just by shopping at the farmers markets and giving vegetables and fruits the center stage, I found myself naturally cutting out animal products—and I felt so much better.

I soon realized that this was it. This was what I wanted to do for the rest of my life. I'd gone on a soul-searching quest, and I'd landed in the kitchen, surrounded by plants. I couldn't wait to learn more. Chefs and cooks would become my teachers and the kitchen would become my classroom.

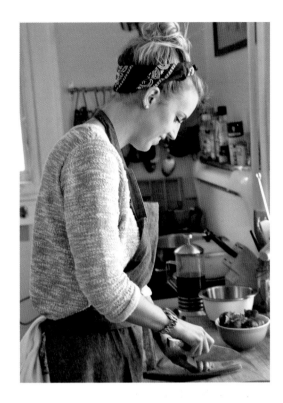

NOM YOURSELF: THE BEGINNING

Filled with love of everything plant-based, plus my growing love of photography, I started a new Instagram, just for my food photos. At this point, Spencer, my nannying charge, started each day wearing a bib illustrating a peanut butter and jelly sandwich, with the words "nom, nom, nom"—a phrase that describes the pleasures of eating, and one we can all relate to. But I wanted to get across the you-can-do-it-too feeling that I'd been trying to spread among my friends and family. So, I came up with Nom Yourself. It was also my own way of saying "calm yourself." My hopes for the account were simple. I wanted to connect with like-minded people

on a culinary journey of eating and cooking a plant-based diet, to inspire those who hadn't even thought of veganism as an option, and to start a kind of "food diary" of my life in the kitchen.

During the next few months as the account started to take off, "Nom Yourself" took on a new meaning: you are what you eat. Simple and true. And I would soon find that this was a message that appealed to many, many people. After mere days, it turned out that thousands of people were instantly interested in what I was doing with vegetables. People started asking for recipes. *Me? Recipes?* I would think, *You do know I was burning sweet potatoes just a couple months ago, right?* But that was the whole point. There were thousands of people in the same exact place I was, just trying to figure out what to do in their kitchens.

Besieged by recipe requests and eager to help my followers out, I taught myself to code websites and started nomyourself.com to share recipes, tips, and

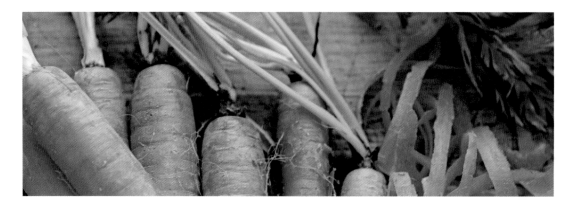

thoughts with those who were so graciously supporting and following my journey into the culinary and
vegan world. I also reached out to interview vegans
from all walks of life, to see how they handled the
challenges and opportunities of a plant-based life. I
knew my story wasn't necessarily a universal one, so I
wanted people exploring a vegan lifestyle to have a
resource where they could come and find someone
like them who was loving veganism. I started
e-mailing people: Chad Sarno, a culinary educator
and chef; Brendan Brazier, an author and formulator
of Vega; Mike Zigomanis, a professional hockey
player; Kimmy McAtee, vice president of marketing
for Keep A Breast, a foundation for breast cancer
awareness; Toby Morse, singer of H2O and founder of
One Life One Chance; Stephanie Fryslie, owner and
shoemaker of Nicora Johns. I interviewed them about
their stories and their journeys to becoming vegan,
and I posted those interviews on the site to encourage
would-be vegans to take the plunge. The World Wide
Web allowed me to form friendships with creative and
motivated individuals who were pushing themselves
to be the best they could possibly be, just like I was.

As I became more and more knowledgeable about
vegan lifestyles, my passion continued to grow.
Endless possibilities unfolded before me, and I
received countless signs that this was the right move
for me. Early in 2014, superstar singer-songwriter Ellie
Goulding tweeted "that looks delicious" at one of my
photos. She's since become an incredible supporter of
Nom Yourself, and our first tentative tweets and

comments have blossomed into a genuine friendship
IRL (in real life, as they say). Later that year, I was
lucky enough to connect with Jeremy Piven on Twitter.
He was a stranger to me at that point, but when we
discovered that we had both eaten at the same
restaurant, he sent me a message stating that he was
interested in talking about a plant-based diet. We met
up to discuss it, and by the end of the meeting we'd
determined that I would become his personal chef that
week and cater for him while he filmed the *Entourage*
movie. The process of cooking for someone who is
utterly dependent on you for health and wellness is an
incredibly amazing feeling, and it gave me a great
sense of fulfillment. My catering career has pro-
gressed from there, as has my friendship with Jeremy.

So I guess you could say I've been lucky—and you
could also say that social media has contributed in
large part to where I am today. I can promise you right
now, I'm never going to stop posting drool-worthy
photos of delicious, decadent vegan sandwiches, and I
think the world will be a better place because of it.

I'm writing to you now from Baltimore. Yes, I'm
back in the city I love, the place where it all began. I'm
cooking in that gorgeous open kitchen, lighting my
oven with a match, shopping at the Waverly Farmers
Market, and writing this cookbook for you with my
whole heart and soul. These recipes are my journey.
They represent all the good times and delicious meals
I've made, plus the wonderful blunders I've made
along the way, each of which taught me something
new. So from my kitchen to yours: enjoy.

THE ESSENTIALS:
STOCKING YOUR KITCHEN AND GETTING STARTED

I'VE NEVER BEEN A HUGE FAN OF GROCERY LISTS. When I do make them I almost never stick to them because I like to venture into the unknown and buy produce that I can't pronounce. This allows me to get more creative in the kitchen and taste new things. That said, it's important to have a few essential staples in your pantry at all times, so that you can actually turn your delicious new produce into edible meals that you enjoy. Below is a list of items I always keep on hand.

> Keep in mind that shopping seasonally and locally is important, both to get the best-tasting produce for your dishes and to support your local agriculture. Look for farmers markets or community supported agriculture (CSA) in your area.

DAIRY SUBSTITUTES

Nondairy Milk (Almond, Soy, Coconut, Rice, Hemp, Whichever You Prefer): Make your own (see pages 16–17), or buy brands such as Califia Farms, Almond Breeze, or Silk, which usually offer various options, such as sweetened, vanilla, and more. I prefer to buy unsweetened original milks so I can use them for a wide variety of recipes. Then I'll add additional sweetness with maple syrup and flavor them with vanilla extract as needed.

Vegan Butter: Chances are you may already buy vegan butter, even if you aren't vegan already! Vegetable-based margarine has become a huge part of the buttery spread market. You can find brands such as Earth Balance at your local grocery store.

Canned Coconut Cream: I almost always use canned coconut purely for the fat it contains. It is great for whipped cream, sour cream, thick sauces, and dressings. Then I use the coconut milk left over in the can for my smoothie the next day.

PANTRY STAPLES

Baking Powder: I've found it doesn't truly matter which baking powder you use, as long as it's stored correctly. Over time baking powder will degrade, especially in humid environments, so once you purchase your baking powder, be sure to transfer it to an airtight jar and keep it in a cool environment.

Baking Soda: Baking soda is not just that orange box you put in the fridge to keep things smelling fresh. It's also a key ingredient in a lot of cakes and batters, as you'll see in the recipes to come. My favorite brand for baking is Bob's Red Mill Baking Soda.

Incidentally, baking soda is also a great natural way to clean your kitchen. Just sprinkle some on your countertops, spray with equal parts water and white distilled vinegar, and scrub!

Raw Nuts: High in protein, nuts are perfect to snack on. They are also really good to have when making thick nondairy sauces and nondairy milks. I usually keep raw unsalted almonds, cashews, walnuts, and pine nuts around. These guys can get pretty expensive, so I usually wait until a sale and try not to over-snack on them.

Nut Butter (Almond, Cashew, Peanut): If you don't have time to make your own nut butter, store-bought can be fine as well, but depending on the brand can also be full of additives. So if you're going with store-bought, stick with a nut butter that has the least amount of ingredients, and preferably just one: nuts!

Garlic Cloves: I use garlic in a lot of dishes, so I tend to pick up one or two bulbs just to have on hand any time I visit the market. Garlic does go bad, though, so before you use them, check to make sure that the cloves are not dry or mushy. It's okay if the garlic has sprouted a bit (you'll know when you see the little green stem showing); just be sure to remove the sprout before use.

Ground Black Pepper: If you can get whole black pepper and grind the peppercorns yourself with a spice grinder, that would be ideal. Ground black pepper is completely fine, though, if you don't have the time or equipment to grind your own pepper.

Dried Herbs and Spices (Parsley, Basil, Chives, Oregano, Paprika): Spices and herbs are always best when fresh. You can easily grow them in your kitchen, but I understand that not everyone has the time to grow their own herbs. I like to keep my cupboard stocked with different spices and dried herbs to try. The ones I use the most are parsley, basil, chives, oregano, paprika, chili powder, and thyme. I usually like to collect dried herbs and spices to try out new flavor profiles. It's always fun to try out new herbs and spices, and the reality is that sometimes they aren't available in their fresh form.

Organic Ground Cinnamon: I love cinnamon. That's actually an understatement. I'm obsessed with cinnamon. I use it in almost every baked good I make, as well as in chilies, soups, and marinades. Nutmeg is also great to have on hand, but I don't use it as much as I use cinnamon.

Flaxseed Meal: You can absolutely buy whole flaxseeds and grind them yourself. However, for convenience, I like to buy Bob's Red Mill Flaxseed Meal. You can use flaxseed meal as an egg replacement in a lot of baking. You can put it in your granola, cereals, and breakfast bars to add fiber to your diet as well.

Chia Seeds: One of the greatest benefits of chia seeds is omega-3. Mama Chia is the chia seed brand I prefer, and it is available in most supermarkets. I don't use chia seeds on a daily basis, but I find myself reaching for them more and more in the kitchen. I like to sneak a tablespoon into sauces to bring another texture element to a dish. You can also simply mix 3 tablespoons of chia seeds with ⅓ cup nondairy milk, a dash of cinnamon, and a drop of vanilla to make a delicious chia seed pudding.

Hemp Seeds/Powder: Hemp seeds and powder are a great source of protein. So, as with chia seeds, I try to incorporate them wherever I can, usually in baked goods or smoothies.

Liquid Aminos, Soy Sauce, and Tamari: I usually have all three in my cupboard, but I tend to gravitate more toward tamari because it is thicker and great for marinades. Bragg Liquid Aminos is my second choice if I am out of tamari. I rarely use soy sauce because most store-bought soy sauce has a very high sodium content.

Unbleached All-Purpose Flour (Gluten-Free, If You'd Like): Always have a bag of flour in your cupboard. My favorite flour is King Arthur Unbleached All-Purpose Flour, or the whole-wheat version. When I'm looking for a gluten-free option, Bob's Red Mill makes a coconut flour perfect for baking, although not necessarily great for breading. For cooking gluten-free savory dishes, I usually go with Bob's Red Mill Gluten-Free Flour.

PROTEIN ALTERNATIVES

Organic Block Tofu: There are many different types of tofu, including soft, medium, firm, and extra firm. I use extra-firm tofu in most of my recipes that call for cooked tofu. It is the most versatile.

Organic Silken Tofu: Silken tofu is unpressed tofu, so it keeps its water content. It is perfect for sauces, dips, or spreads you would like to keep thick but smooth. It's also terrific for cheesecakes.

Tempeh: Tempeh has a grainy texture that people either love or hate. I use tempeh as an alternative to bacon because when you marinate it, it takes on the flavor of the marinade well, and it also gets crispy when you cook it.

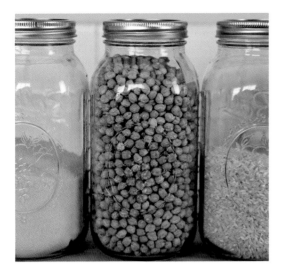

Legumes: Beans, peas, and lentils are a great source of protein and normally have a long shelf life. While I recommend that you purchase bagged, uncooked legumes and soak them, using canned is fine as long as you choose organic. I like to keep black beans, kidney beans, cannellini beans, lentils, chickpeas, and edamame in my cupboard.

TVP: TVP is short for textured vegetable protein. I use Bob's Red Mill TVP as a beef alternative in dishes such as chili, lasagna, or wherever I would normally use beef.

Mock Meats: If you've been past the "Healthy Alternatives" aisle in the freezer section, you've likely seen mock meats such as Gardein, Morning Star, and Beyond Meat. They are a great option if you are transitioning into a vegan lifestyle. These mock meats helped me when I first started eating a plant-based diet.

> Although dry herbs get the job done, it's always great to have fresh herbs such as basil, rosemary, thyme, and sage on hand. If you can grow them in your kitchen, that's one less thing on your grocery list! And you know how I feel about grocery lists. . . .

SWEETENERS

Pure Maple Syrup: Make sure you buy pure maple syrup. A lot of syrups in the supermarket have additives in them that take away from their taste and nutritional value. Maple syrup is defined by four grades: Vermont Fancy, Grade A Medium Amber, Grade A Dark Amber, and Grade B. In pure form, each of these syrups has the same nutritional value, as none of them is refined. So it really is all about preference. I tend to lean more toward Grade B syrup because I like its dark color and rich flavor.

Organic Brown Sugar: Both light brown and dark brown sugar are great to have on hand. The only difference between light brown and dark brown sugar is the amount of molasses each one contains. Dark brown sugar has a bit more of a toffee taste, whereas light brown sugar has a less intense flavor.

Organic Powdered/Confectioners' Sugar: Don't be confused by the words "powdered" and "confectioners.'" They are the exact same thing. It is just sugar that is processed multiple times to make a powder. This is a great sugar to have on hand for finishing pastries as well as making glazes and frosting.

Dates: If you're trying to stay away from refined sugars, dates are a great alternative. You can use them to add sweetness to your smoothies, eat them raw, or use them as a refined sugar alternative in baked goods. I use six blended dates for every cup of sugar.

Agave Nectar: I try to stay away from agave nectar as a sweetener because of its high fructose content, but I keep it in my cupboard to use occasionally when dates wouldn't be an acceptable substitute, such as in sauces.

VINEGARS

Apple Cider Vinegar: Even if you're not one of those people who does a shot of the stuff every day, apple cider vinegar is essential in any kitchen for baking, vinaigrettes, and any number of delectable uses. I've found that Bragg makes the most natural apple cider vinegar. A few notes on how good cider vinegar should look: you want it to be cloudy. You'll also see some white substance sitting on the bottom of the jar or bottle; this is called the mother. Don't worry, you want this in there. Stay away from any filtered brands.

White Wine Vinegar: When you see this called for in recipes, it's possible that you'll think *Can't I just use white vinegar?* Confession: I tried that when I first started cooking. And I can tell you for sure: the answer is *no*. White wine vinegar is the best cooking vinegar because it is made from the fermentation of white wine. It keeps the flavor you want while still giving you the acid you need. Conversely, white (distilled) vinegar has a strong acidic taste, which you do not want in your food.

Red Wine Vinegar: Red wine vinegar is perfect for reductions and sauces and is great for pickling as well.

Balsamic Vinegar: I use balsamic vinegar for reductions and sauces, but mostly I like to drizzle it on salad with a little extra-virgin olive oil and lemon juice. It makes the perfect salad dressing all on its own when you don't have time to make homemade dressing.

OILS AND SALTS, AND HOW TO USE THEM

The more you learn about how food is made, the more you'll want to learn how to use your ingredients properly. Before I knew what I was doing in the kitchen, I would use ingredients in all the wrong ways, particularly salt and oil. I used canola oil all the time, put fleur de sel in baking recipes, and fried things in olive oil. To keep you from making my mistakes, I've put together a small guide on how to use these important basic ingredients.

If you're trying to minimize oil in your diet, don't fear! You can absolutely substitute vegetable broth for oil in many of my recipes.

OIL

Every oil has a different smoke point, which is the temperature at which the oil starts to smoke, and the smoke points for a given type of oil will also vary depending on how it's been produced and handled before it reaches your shelf. The label on the bottle will usually be helpful in determining the smoke point, but generally, the more refined an oil is, the higher the smoke point will be.

Whatever the smoke point is for a given oil, you don't want to exceed this temperature. Make sure to consult this section closely in order to avoid burning anything (and to prevent any fires in the kitchen).

EXTRA-VIRGIN OLIVE OIL
Smoke Point: Low
When I first started cooking, I used extra-virgin olive oil to sauté everything. Nine times out of ten my food would end up burned, and I didn't understand why. I had been told that extra-virgin olive oil was healthy for you, so if I was going to cook with oil, that's what I was using. Finally I learned that the health benefits apply when you don't *cook* the olive oil. While extra-virgin olive oil is extremely nutrient-dense, it loses its nutrients and flavor when it's heated. Now, I use EVOO for dipping with fresh herbs, drizzling over a salad, or mixing into bruschetta. Note that EVOO is not to be confused with refined olive oil, which has a much higher smoke point.

CANOLA OIL
Smoke Point: Medium
I'm including this on the list to educate you, but if possible, stay away from canola oil. A lot of people think that "canola" is a plant. It is actually a contrac-

tion of Canada Oil, Low Acid. Ninety percent of canola oil is made from genetically modified rapeseed. It doesn't have any nutritional benefits.

SESAME OIL
Smoke Point: Medium
The most common sesame oils used and sold in supermarkets are light sesame oil and dark sesame oil, also known as toasted sesame oil. Light sesame oil has a higher smoke point and can be used in deep-frying. Dark sesame oil is the more common household oil and has a lower smoke point. It can be used for stir-fry and in sauces or marinades. Dark sesame oil has a very distinct, strong sesame smell. A couple of drops go a long way.

SAFFLOWER OIL
Smoke Point: Medium
Safflower oil increases adiponectin, which is a protein that helps regulate blood glucose levels and break down fatty acids in your body. For this reason, it is best to use safflower oil in its raw form and not in cooking. I like to use it for vinaigrettes or drizzled on salads with balsamic vinegar.

COCONUT OIL
Smoke Point: Medium-High
Coconut oil comes in two forms, unrefined or "virgin" coconut oil and refined coconut oil. When choosing a coconut oil, keep in mind that they have two different smoke points. Refined oils in general have a higher smoke point. Virgin coconut oil has a smoking point of 350 degrees F, whereas refined coconut oil's smoke point is 450 degrees F.

Coconut oil is the only oil that can retain its nutrients at a medium to high heat, which makes it one of the safest and healthiest oils to use in cooking. I use virgin/unrefined coconut oil for baking and roasting, and refined coconut oil for sautéing.

PEANUT OIL
Smoke Point: High
While peanut oil has no real health benefit when it's heated above 212 degrees F, it is great for deep-frying because it doesn't transfer flavors or absorb the flavor of whatever you're frying, so you can use the same oil to deep-fry multiple ingredients or batches.

AVOCADO OIL
Smoke Point: High
There are two types of avocado oil in stores, unrefined or "virgin" avocado oil and refined avocado oil. Unrefined avocado oil has a smoke point of 480 degrees F. Yes, you read that right. Refined avocado oil's smoke point is even higher: 520 degrees F. With the highest smoke point of any oil, avocado oil, either virgin or refined, is great for pan-frying and searing. It is also great for deep frying, but that's definitely not a cost-efficient use because avocado oil is quite expensive. Still, I love to keep it in my kitchen at all times because I can do pretty much everything with it: bake, deep-fry, sear, roast, sauté—the list goes on!

SALT

Recently I've been trying to minimize the salt in my diet, to let the natural flavor of my food shine through and reduce my sodium intake. I've started replacing salt with extra fresh herbs and lots of garlic. When I do use salt, though, I like to use the best salt for the dish I'm making.

TABLE SALT
Table salt is my least favorite salt to cook with due to its lack of flavor. A large amount of fortified table salt is used in almost all processed foods and it doesn't necessarily add to the flavor. In addition, most table salt has chemical additives and is stripped of its natural minerals during production.

SEA SALT
My top choice of salt to use in the kitchen is sea salt. I like the flavor it brings out in a dish and how it feels in my hands. It's also a great finishing salt for when I don't want to use too much. Sea salt comes in a variety of coarseness grades, so pick your favorite.

One note: Contrary to popular belief, sea salt and table salt have the same basic nutritional value. So it really comes down to preference of flavor.

KOSHER SALT

Did you know that nearly all salt is already kosher? "Kosher salt" is called that because this particular kind of salt is used in the removal of surface blood during the process of making kosher meat, which, if you're reading this book, is probably not how you'll be using it!

Kosher salt is great because it dissolves evenly, which makes it perfect for sauces, baking, and soups. I like to call kosher salt the bona fide table salt, because although kosher salt contains sodium chloride, it does not contain the additives that table salt does.

FLEUR DE SEL

Fleur de sel, which means "flower of salt" in French, is my favorite "special occasion" finishing salt. It's a little more expensive than other salts because of its labor-intensive production process, so I save this salt for my guests of honor in dishes I have not salted much throughout the cooking process. Use it sparingly, but deliciously.

NOM NOTES

You'll see Nom Notes throughout this book to give you tips on the dish at hand, offer ideas on how to make meals not in this book, or help you plate. Think of them as my little thoughts to you while you're cooking. It's always nice to have a little reminder that someone else has made these recipes and knows the struggles and joys of being in the kitchen while making them.

ESSENTIAL EQUIPMENT

I love kitchen gadgets. I'm a sucker for things that are completely useless when it comes to cooking. Or, I should say, I used to be. Once the kitchen became a place I wanted to be in for the greater part of my day, I realized that the clutter of useless machinery had to go. That meant "bye-bye, garlic mincer that had cute little wheels but was a pain to clean." And "so long, ten different cutting boards." (Who needs that many cutting boards?) So I've come up with a list to give you the essentials. Gadgets are fun, but having just the basics really helps you become a better cook because you don't rely on machinery to do it for you.

Stationary Blender: Try not to get lost in the plethora of online reviews over which blender is best. The one you have in your kitchen is probably just fine for now. If you don't own a blender and are looking for a new one, keep in mind that you will use this machine often. If you're just looking for a smoothie maker, I suggest going with the most basic model, but if you want something for more heavy-duty kitchen tasks, you'll need one with a better motor. Don't save a couple bucks now only to end up spending more down the line.

Immersion Blender: I cannot say enough great things about the immersion blender. I was gifted one a couple of years ago and was too intimidated to even think about using it. Then I saw a friend use it to make soup and I was in awe. It's easy to clean and quick to use. Whenever someone asks me what appliance I value most in the kitchen, my answer is always the almighty immersion blender. It is also referred to as a handheld blender or a stick blender.

Food Processor: I rarely used my food processor before becoming vegan. It just collected dust in my cabinet. Then I started making sauces and chopping more solids and I quickly learned the true value of the food processor. I'll tell you honestly: this will be your right-hand man in the kitchen. When you need things chopped, sliced, or blended fast, this is your go-to machine.

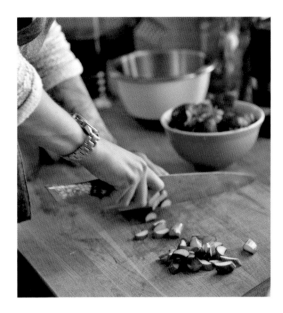
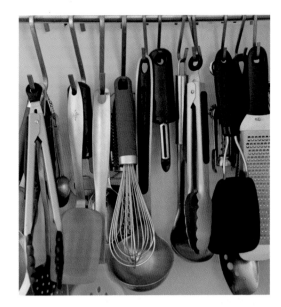

Chef's Knife: They say a knife is an extension of your hand, and it is absolutely true. Especially the chef's knife, or, as some call it, cook's knife, which is a multipurpose and essential tool for chopping vegetables, crushing garlic, dicing fruit, and much, much more. If you use it right, it is *the* most important tool you will use to make food.

Cutting Board: The big debate about cutting boards is whether to go wooden or synthetic. The answer for me is always wood. While synthetic comes in a wide variety of colors and shapes, as well as being very light, it also stains easily and after a while forms grooves that make it difficult to cut on. I prefer wood because it's beautiful and lasts awhile if maintained correctly. Yes, wood cutting boards get wear and tear as well, but that just gives them a little character.

Whisks: It's good to have whisks in a variety of sizes, from large ones for whipping coconut cream to small whisks for stirring sauces. Make sure you get stainless steel, which is easier to clean and more efficient to use.

Spatulas: I have the craziest collection of spatulas, from nylon to stainless steel, large and small, all colors and shapes. Is it really necessary to have all these spatulas? The answer is yes. Each one has its own

purpose. If you use nonstick pans, you should be using only nylon or plastic utensils on them so that you don't damage the coating on the pans. However, if you do not use nonstick pans, metal spatulas are easier and more efficient to use. I have a mix of pans, so having a variety of these utensils is necessary.

Mixing Bowls: Stainless steel is key when you're choosing mixing bowls. Stainless steel bowls are easy to clean and your food won't stick to the sides of them as it would in ceramic or plastic bowls. Plus they're lightweight, which makes it easier to keep the flow of your cooking going. I have three or four mixing bowls of various sizes.

Sieve: A sieve is a wire mesh strainer used to separate liquids from solids. I keep two sizes of sieves in my kitchen—small and large. Each has a handle, as I find handles make a sieve easier to use. They are great for sprinkling confectioners' sugar on dishes as well as straining pulp and/or seeds from juices.

Sauté Pan: A sauté pan has vertical sides and is deeper in depth than a skillet. My sauté pans have always been stainless steel rather than nonstick because when I use my sauté pan, there's usually a good amount of liquid (water or oil) in the pan too, which means no need for nonstick.

Skillet: Also known as a frying pan, a skillet is actually best for sautéing. Sounds crazy, I know. The skillet's slanted sides make it easy to sauté and move ingredients around. However, both the sauté pan and skillet can perform almost all tasks equally. So if you have only one of them on hand, don't stress.

Saucepan: Saucepans come in all sizes, from one pint to four quarts, and it's good to have the different sizes on hand to complete whatever recipe you're making. You want to make sure you have a saucepan with a sturdy handle. I made the mistake of buying a cheap saucepan years ago, and let's just say the handle and pan did not stay together long.

Stockpot: A stockpot is a huge pot with two handles mostly used for cooking a large amount of liquids. However, they have a wide variety of uses: boiling pasta, blanching vegetables, making broth, and much more. A good stockpot should be stainless steel and have sturdy handles. Some handles may have heat protectors on them. If they don't, be sure to use a kitchen towel to lift the pot, as the handles will be hot after cooking.

> Always turn on the radio before you cook. Listening to music has a huge impact on the dishes I make and the mood I am in. It will help get your creative juices flowing and make your imagination run wild. Music will cancel out any thoughts you have about what else you have going on in your life and allow you to have that moment in the kitchen for yourself.

BUY LOCAL PRODUCE

I found my way to a vegan lifestyle and a plant-based diet by learning to eat locally and seasonally, all thanks to my local farmers market. Shopping at Waverly Farmers Market in Baltimore each Saturday morning gave me a sense of real community within a city that I'd previously found intimidating and impersonal. It gave me a chance to talk to farmers and other people at the market about cooking, eating, how amazing last week's arugula was, and what I planned to do with this week's peaches. In the hectic society we live in today, it was nice to take an hour or two out of my weekend to connect with people who were passionate about the same thing I was: food.

I also became about a thousand times healthier as a result of eating local fruits and vegetables. The produce I cooked with each week was organic, non-GMO, packed with nutrients, and had been harvested about twenty minutes from where I lived—sometimes it even came from my own backyard. When produce has to be transported to your local grocery store from thousands of miles away, it loses its nutritional value at a steep rate, so eating local gives you more nutrients, plain and simple.

One thing that a lot of people don't think about: larger companies harvest their fruits and vegetables according to a pre-appointed schedule instead of when they become perfectly ripe. Then they'll treat the produce with ethylene gas to speed up the off-the-vine ripening process and make it look beautiful for you, the consumer. Yuck! The difference between biting into a tomato in a grocery store and a local tomato picked fresh off the vine for its ripeness is incredible.

Sure, GMO foods look beautiful—that's because they're bred to look that way. When you're eating organic, local produce, you'll learn to embrace the bumps and bruises on fruits and vegetables. It gives them character and makes you appreciate that what you're buying is real.

Eating local is what's best for you and for your community. It's undeniable. So I encourage you to find a farmers market or CSA in your neighborhood, and always go there before you head to the grocery store. And try a new vegetable! There are so many kinds of veggies out there—things you don't even know exist. Just the other day I cooked fresh Jerusalem artichokes for the first time after hearing a farmer raving about how perfect they are this time of year. Explore! Have fun with your food.

FOOD IS ART!

Vegan food used to be stigmatized as bland and boring—the opposite of the beautiful gourmet food consumed by the carnivores of the world. But no more! The world has seen the light, and more and more chefs have begun celebrating vegetables as a main dish, paving the way for veganism to enter the world of upscale cuisine. So become an artist! Let the plate be your canvas and create an edible painting. Plant-based food doesn't have to be a pile of rice and beans or a bunch of chopped lettuce.

HERE ARE SOME TIPS FOR PREPARING BEAUTIFUL DISHES

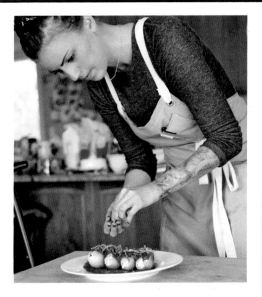

USE WHITE PLATES
Using colored or patterned plates takes away from the beautiful colors and textures that vegetables bring to a dish. White plates make your food pop!

FOLLOW THE RAINBOW RULE
Make sure your plate has lots of color. For example, if you're going to make Half-Baked Macaroni and Cheese (page 111), pair it with some bright green sautéed Swiss chard and luscious maroon roasted beets.

SAUCE IT FIRST
If you take the time to carefully plate your dish or put your salad into a food stacker, the last thing you want is for the weight of the sauce or dressing to ruin your creation. So, before you plate, take a spoon and either make a circle of sauce around the edge of the plate or drizzle the sauce in a zigzag motion across the plate, and then place your dish in the center. Placing food on top of the sauce allows you to showcase the beauty of the main dish while using the sauce to create another artistic element on the plate.

USE THESE SIMPLE TOOLS TO UP YOUR GAME
Don't worry, you don't need any fancy new chef ware to make your dishes look like perfection. There are only three plating tools you need to make your recipes look like every photo in this book: squeeze bottles, for drizzling sauces; food stackers, to make food nice and clean; and last, but not least, a good chef's knife. Learning how to use a chef's knife properly will help your final dishes' appearance tremendously. Get creative on the shape of your ingredients by varying how you cut them.

Honorable mention: kitchen tweezers. When you are garnishing or dealing with delicate details as you plate, tweezers can sometimes make or break the final outcome. They are fairly cheap and a great investment for your plating skills.

GARNISH
To make your finished dish look really elegant, garnish it with a fresh sprig of an herb (like rosemary or sage) or spice or a citrus rind. It's like when a concession stand attendant puts a little extra vegan butter on your popcorn. Sure, it's not strictly necessary, but it can make a world of difference.

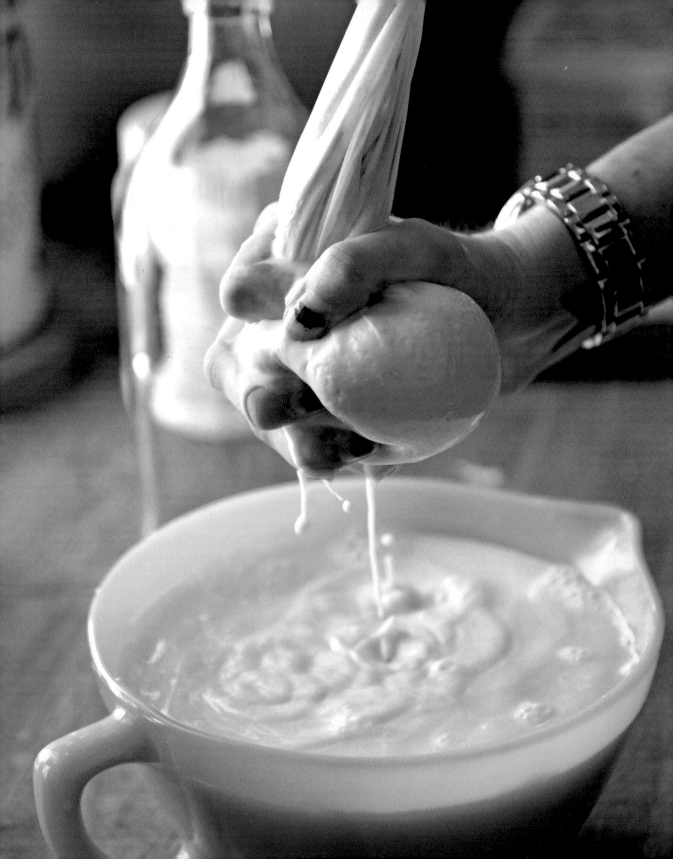

HOMEMADE STAPLES

In the recipes in this book, you'll see callouts for things such as almond milk, cashew cream, and vegan sour cream quite often. You can buy premade from companies like Tofutti, Silk, and others, but when I have the time I like to make my own so I can have total control over what goes in. These recipes are a snap to pull together in a blender (Vitamix is my favorite, but don't fret if you don't have one—a standard blender works just as well).

ALMOND MILK

MAKES ABOUT 3 CUPS OF ALMOND MILK

1 cup raw unsalted almonds, soaked overnight
3 cups water
½ teaspoon vanilla extract (optional)

1. Drain the soaked almonds and place them in a blender with the water. Add the vanilla now, if using.

2. Blend on high for 1 minute.

3. Pour the almond milk into a sieve or cheesecloth over a bowl. Strain the liquid into the bowl and discard the solids left over.

4. Transfer the almond milk to a jar or use right away. It keeps for about 1 week in the refrigerator.

Feel free to add the vanilla if you like your almond milk a little sweeter. I usually skip it in order to make sure I can use my almond milk in any kind of recipe, not just a sweet one.

CASHEW CREAM

MAKES ABOUT 2 CUPS OF CASHEW CREAM

2 cups raw unsalted cashews, soaked overnight
1 tablespoon lemon juice
½ cup water

1. Drain the soaked cashews and place them in a blender with the lemon juice and water.

2. Blend on high for 1 minute or until creamy. Feel free to add more water, one tablespoon at a time, if you prefer a thinner consistency.

3. Transfer the cashew cream to a jar or use right away. It keeps for up to 5 days in the refrigerator.

CASHEW CREAM CHEESE

MAKES ABOUT 2 CUPS OF CASHEW CREAM CHEESE

2 cups raw unsalted cashews, soaked overnight
½ cup water
2 tablespoons organic freshly squeezed lemon juice
1 tablespoon organic apple cider vinegar
1 teaspoon fine sea salt or kosher salt

1. Drain the soaked cashews and place them in a blender with the water, lemon juice, apple cider vinegar, and sea salt.

2. Blend on high in 10-second intervals until thick and creamy. Be sure to scrape down the sides of the blender after every 10-second interval.

3. Transfer the cashew cream cheese to a jar or use right away. It keeps for up to 1 week in the refrigerator.

COCONUT MILK

MAKES ABOUT 4 CUPS OF COCONUT MILK

3 cups water
1½ cups dried coconut chips or flakes

1. Heat the water in a small saucepan over high heat until it just starts to boil. Remove the pan from the heat.

2. Place the coconut chips in a blender. Pour the water over the coconut and blend on high for 2 minutes.

3. Pour the blended mixture into a sieve or cheesecloth over a bowl. Strain the liquid into the bowl and discard the solids left over.

4. Transfer the coconut milk to a jar or use right away. It keeps for up to 3 days in the refrigerator.

COCONUT SOUR CREAM

MAKES ABOUT 1 CUP OF COCONUT SOUR CREAM

1 cup coconut cream, refrigerated
1½ tablespoons organic apple cider vinegar
1 tablespoon freshly squeezed lemon juice
⅛ teaspoon kosher salt

1. Whisk the coconut cream, apple cider vinegar, lemon juice, and kosher salt together in a medium bowl.

2. Transfer the coconut sour cream to a jar or use right away. It keeps for up to 3 days in the refrigerator.

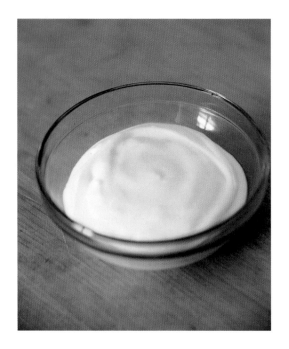

18

MAKING YOUR OWN VEGETABLE BROTH

Tired of buying vegetable broth that is saltier than the sea? Me, too. By the time I'd been cooking for a few months, I had produced a lot of vegetable scraps—onion peels, carrot heads, celery greens, that last quarter bunch of parsley . . . I composted them faithfully, but I always wished I could use them for something else as well. And now I can!

Once you've tried this recipe for the first time, you'll look forward to having those leftover veggie scraps. Just throw them into a ziplock bag and toss them in the freezer, and once the bag is full, whip up this broth and use it in your next soup. And of course, feel very free to modify this recipe—these are basic guidelines for what makes a good broth, but you can absolutely swap, add, or remove ingredients based on what you have left over in your kitchen.

MAKES 2 QUARTS OF BROTH

1 large onion, chopped
2 carrots, chopped
2 stalks celery, chopped
½ cup white button mushrooms, washed and
  chopped
1 parsnip, chopped
4 cloves garlic, whole
1 bunch of fresh flat-leaf parsley
2 bay leaves
1 tablespoon liquid aminos or soy sauce
8 cups water
Salt and freshly ground black pepper to taste

1. Place the onion, carrots, celery, mushrooms, parsnip, garlic, parsley, bay leaves, liquid aminos, water, and salt and pepper in a large pot and bring to a boil.

2. Place the lid on the pot and reduce the heat to medium-low. Let simmer for 1 hour.

3. Place a strainer over a large bowl and pour the broth, vegetables, and herbs into the strainer, collecting the broth in the bowl below.

4. Discard the vegetables and herbs.

5. If you like your broth extra-smooth, pour it through cheesecloth into another bowl to remove any small solids.

6. Use the broth right away, or transfer it to a jar, let it cool to room temperature, cover it with an airtight lid, and place it into the refrigerator for up to 5 days. Or freeze it in a ziplock bag to use within the next 3 months.

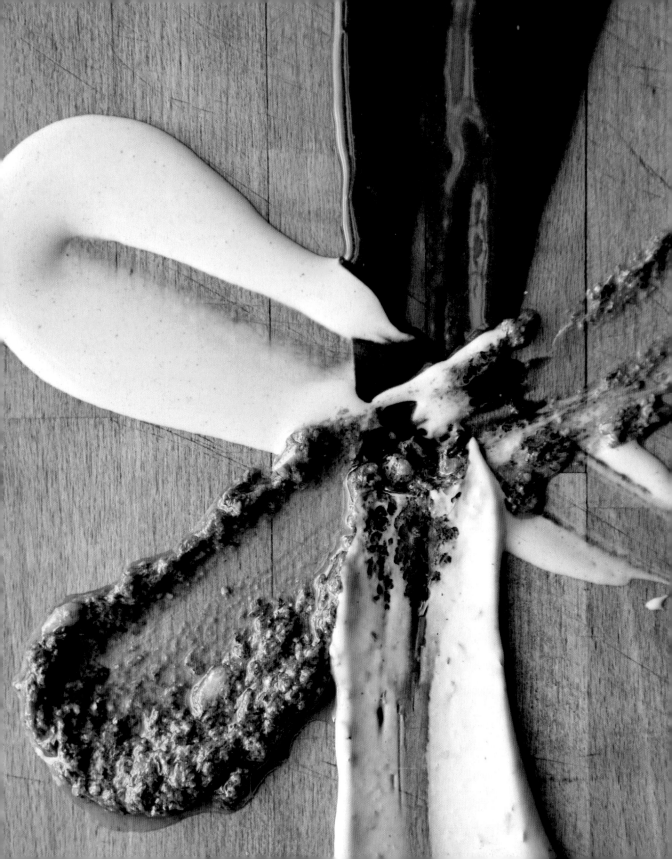

SAUCES, DIPS & DRESSINGS

A good dressing can change the way you look at a salad. It will take it from mediocre to extraordinary by bringing out the natural tastes of an ingredient and combining it with perfectly complementary spices and a creamy texture.

Or picture this: you've come to the end of your farmers market bounty, and all you have left in your fridge is one basic, bland ingredient. Celery. Tofu. Cauliflower. Whatever it is, pair it with a great sauce, and suddenly you've got yourself a magical meal!

Need to satisfy a sweet tooth? You can't go wrong with my vegan versions of caramel sauce and chocolate sauce in this chapter. Drizzle them over fruit, vegan ice cream, pies, cakes, and more. A delicious indulgence!

In this chapter, you'll find recipes for dressings and sauces both basic and a little more advanced. Making these recipes helped me a lot, especially when I first started eating plant-based. Try to make two or three of these recipes ahead each week so your prep for each meal is easier and you can focus on cooking the main ingredients.

KALE PESTO

I love pesto. If I had to choose one thing to eat for the rest of my life, it would be pesto. So I came up with a recipe to make that gallon of pesto that my dreams are made of just a little bit more nutritious. Kale has a sweet and bitter taste that pairs magically with a good extra-virgin olive oil. Enjoy this pesto as a dipping sauce, on pasta, or on a sandwich. I've also been known to just eat it with a spoon.

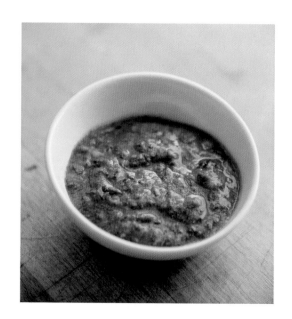

MAKES 1 CUP OF PESTO

2 cups chopped kale leaves
½ cup fresh basil leaves
2 tablespoons pine nuts, toasted
¼ cup extra-virgin olive oil
4 cloves garlic
1 teaspoon onion powder
1 teaspoon nutritional yeast
1 teaspoon sea salt

1. In a blender, add the kale, basil, and pine nuts. Pulse until the ingredients are finely chopped.

2. Add the extra-virgin olive oil, garlic, onion powder, nutritional yeast, and sea salt. Pulse until well combined.

3. Place in a glass jar and store in the refrigerator for up to 14 days.

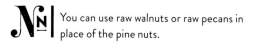 You can use raw walnuts or raw pecans in place of the pine nuts.

SWEET CILANTRO CHILI SAUCE

I was visiting Toronto, Canada, one time and got this tangy fresh chili sauce from a hole-in-the-wall burger joint. I know, burger joint and cilantro chili sauce? You'd think they don't go together, but they do. If you're into sweet and spicy (mostly spicy) sauces, this recipe is for you. Sweet Cilantro Chili Sauce goes great on tacos and banh mi, or tossed with roasted vegetables.

MAKES 4 SERVINGS OR ABOUT 1 CUP OF SAUCE

¼ cup chili sauce
⅓ cup rice vinegar
½ cup organic brown sugar
1½ teaspoons ground ginger
1 teaspoon garlic powder
¼ cup organic ketchup
2 tablespoons cornstarch
¼ cup cold water
½ teaspoon red pepper flakes

1. In a small saucepan, mix the chili sauce, rice vinegar, brown sugar, ginger, garlic powder, and ketchup together.

2. Bring the mixture to a boil over high heat.

3. Meanwhile, in a small bowl, mix the cornstarch and water together.

4. Stir the cornstarch mixture into the chili sauce mixture. Reduce the heat to low and bring to a simmer. Cook for 2 to 3 minutes, until the sauce thickens.

5. Remove the pan from the heat and let the sauce cool for 5 minutes before serving.

SPICY CILANTRO PEANUT SAUCE

The key to a good peanut sauce is the consistency—it shouldn't be too thick or too runny. In order to find the right balance, start with a thick sauce, and then add more liquids as needed. Also, feel free to add more water if you've mixed the peanut butter too much. It will absorb the liquids quickly. Make this sauce at the beginning of the week, and you'll be able to have a delicious side dish ready in just minutes every night by using a tablespoon or two of it on top of steamed veggies.

MAKES 4 SERVINGS OR ABOUT 2/3 CUP OF SAUCE

½ cup creamy peanut butter
¼ cup rice vinegar
¼ cup freshly squeezed lime juice
3 tablespoons coconut oil
1 tablespoon soy sauce
3 tablespoons blue agave nectar
½ tablespoon grated fresh ginger
½ teaspoon chili sauce
¼ cup finely chopped fresh cilantro leaves

1. In the bowl of a food processor, blend the peanut butter, rice vinegar, lime juice, coconut oil, soy sauce, agave, ginger, and chili sauce until fully combined.

2. Add the cilantro and pulse two or three times.

3. Use immediately or pour into a storage jar and refrigerate for up to 1 week.

COCONUT MUSHROOM GRAVY

There is nothing more comforting than pouring a heap of gravy over some mashed potatoes. For me, they go together like macaroni and cheese. In this recipe I exchange the animal fat that is traditionally used in gravy with the plant-based fat of coconut (I warned you I love coconut fat). Nothing makes people feel more at home than gravy, and this coconut mushroom version is a great addition to any table.

MAKES 4 SERVINGS OR ABOUT 2 CUPS OF GRAVY

¼ cup vegan butter
1½ cups baby bella mushrooms, washed and sliced
1 small onion, chopped
3 cloves garlic, diced
2 cups Vegetable Broth (page 19)
1 cup canned coconut milk
3 tablespoons nutritional yeast
2 tablespoons chopped fresh basil
1 teaspoon chopped fresh thyme
1 teaspoon plus a pinch kosher salt
2 tablespoons sifted unbleached all-purpose flour

1. In a large skillet, heat the vegan butter over medium heat.

2. Once the vegan butter is hot, add the mushrooms, onion, and garlic and sauté for about 4 minutes, until the onion and mushrooms are tender.

3. Add the vegetable broth, coconut milk, nutritional yeast, basil, thyme, and a pinch of salt and bring to a boil.

4. Add the flour and the remaining 1 teaspoon salt. Reduce the heat to a simmer and cook for another 10 minutes, stirring occasionally.

5. Remove the skillet from the heat and let it sit, covered, for about 5 minutes, until the sauce thickens.

 Enjoy over mashed potatoes, seitan loaf, or even just plain pasta. Toss in some roasted veggies and you've got dinner!

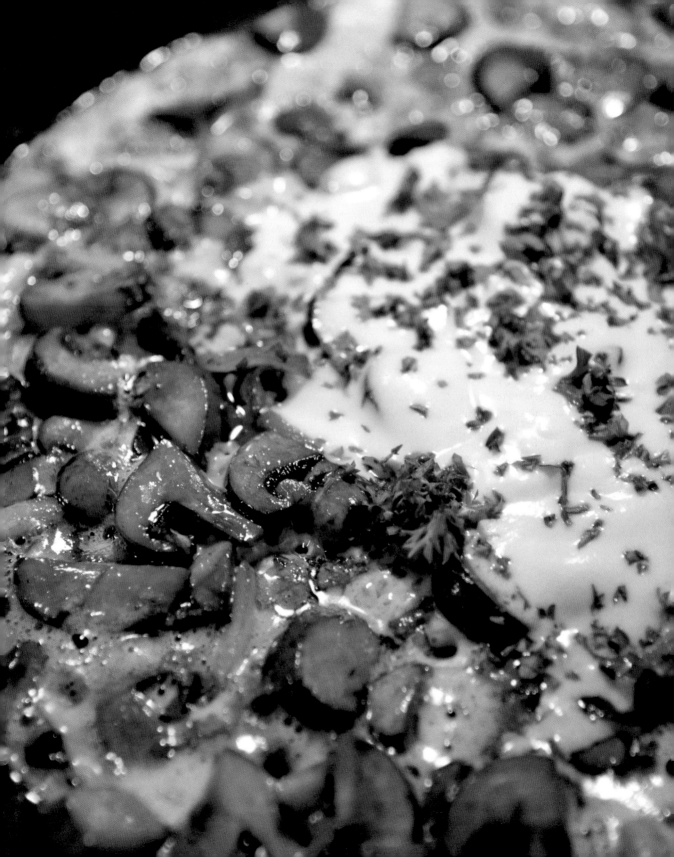

HERB CASHEW CREAM

If you're looking for a cheese-spread fix, this recipe is for you. It's perfect on crostini, as a dip, or even mixed in with your favorite pasta. Feel free to substitute your favorite herbs or whatever you have in your kitchen or garden.

MAKES 10 SERVINGS OR 3 CUPS OF CASHEW CREAM

1½ cups unsalted raw cashews
3 cups water
Freshly squeezed juice of ½ large lemon
1 tablespoon finely chopped fresh basil
1 teaspoon finely chopped fresh rosemary
2 cloves garlic, roasted and minced
½ teaspoon sea salt

1. Soak the cashews in 2 cups of the water for at least 4 hours or overnight.

2. Drain and rinse the cashews.

3. In a blender, blend the cashews, the remaining 1 cup water, and the lemon juice until thick and smooth.

4. Pour the cashew mixture into a medium bowl and mix in the basil, rosemary, garlic, and sea salt until well combined.

5. Spread on toast, use on macaroni, or dab on a bowl of tomatoes and enjoy!

NN Do not mix your fresh herbs with the cashew cream in the blender, or your cream will turn green. You want nice fresh white cream to bring out the herbs. You can refrigerate the cashew cream for up to 5 days, so it's great to make some for the whole week.

ALMOND CHEESE SAUCE

This obviously is not dairy cheese, because well . . . this is a vegan cookbook. Though, if you taste this sauce and have no idea it's milk-free, then I've done my job right. This will satisfy the pickiest mac and cheese enthusiasts, dairy lovers, and those vegans who don't like vegan cheese. It is simple and amazing!

MAKES 4 SERVINGS OR 1½ CUPS OF SAUCE

¼ cup vegan butter
1 cup unsweetened almond milk
2 cups vegan shredded cheese
1 teaspoon garlic powder
1 teaspoon onion powder
¼ teaspoon sea salt

1. In a medium saucepan, melt the vegan butter in the almond milk over medium heat.

2. Once the vegan butter has melted, add the vegan cheese, garlic powder, onion powder, and sea salt.

3. Stir occasionally so that the vegan cheese does not stick to the bottom of the pan.

4. Cook for 10 minutes. Remove from the heat and stir until smooth and thick.

N | Put the sauce in the fridge and let it cool for 20 minutes, then smear on bread and grill for an epic grilled cheese, or toss on some pasta for an easy mac and cheese.

MILLION ISLAND DRESSING

Cheesy name for a fresh take on Thousand Island dressing? Maybe, but I feel it's warranted. Growing up, Thousand Island dressing was a staple in our household. Sandwiches weren't complete until they'd been loaded with the creamy relish dressing. For this version, I've cut out the dairy and taken the whole shebang to a spicier level. Instead of using traditional ketchup, I like to use chili sauce. Poppa Mattern approves.

MAKES 5 SERVINGS OR ABOUT 1 CUP OF DRESSING

1 cup vegan mayonnaise
2 tablespoons chili sauce
1 tablespoon sweet pickle relish
½ small onion, minced
1 teaspoon garlic powder
Freshly ground black pepper to taste

1. Mix the vegan mayonnaise, chili sauce, pickle relish, onion, garlic powder, and pepper in a small bowl.

2. Pour the dressing into an easy-pour bottle and let it chill in the refrigerator for 4 hours or until ready to use.

N | When using heavy dressings, always remember to put it on the plate first instead of drizzling it on top so you don't weigh down your greens and so you can showcase them beautifully on your plate.

CAESAR DRESSING

Plant-based creamy dressings are hard to come by, especially a good Caesar salad dressing. The Dijon mustard in this recipe brings out that special tang you look for in a Caesar dressing. Just grill some romaine halves and top with capers, croutons, and thinly sliced cucumbers, and you've got a pretty magical lunchtime meal!

MAKES ABOUT 1½ CUPS OF DRESSING

1 cup vegan sour cream
⅓ cup vegan mayonnaise
3 tablespoons freshly squeezed lemon juice
1 tablespoon tahini powder
½ teaspoon Dijon mustard, plus more to taste
½ teaspoon garlic powder
1 teaspoon sea salt
¼ teaspoon freshly ground black pepper

1. Mix the vegan sour cream, vegan mayonnaise, lemon juice, tahini powder, mustard, garlic powder, sea salt, and pepper in a medium bowl.

2. Add a little more Dijon mustard if you want some more tang in your dressing.

3. Pour the dressing into an easy-pour bottle and let it chill in the refrigerator for 4 hours or until ready to use.

BUTTERMILK RANCH DIP

I've been known to eat a lot more ranch dip than one should probably consume. I mean, it's pretty much the best dressing, and it goes great on everything. I dip my pizza, sandwiches, Fried Eggplant Sticks (page 79), and cauliflower buffalo bites in it. Oh yeah, and sometimes I pour it on salad. Sometimes.

**MAKES A LITTLE MORE THAN
2 CUPS OF RANCH DIP**

1½ cups vegan mayonnaise
½ teaspoon garlic powder
½ teaspoon onion powder
¼ teaspoon freshly ground black pepper
2 teaspoons dried parsley
⅓ cup unsweetened almond milk
1 teaspoon organic apple cider vinegar

1. Whisk the vegan mayonnaise, garlic powder, onion powder, pepper, parsley, almond milk, and apple cider vinegar in a medium bowl.

2. If the dip is too thin, add more vegan mayonnaise to make it your preferred consistency.

 Two words: Buffalo Cauliflower. Check it out in Buffalo Cauliflower Kale Salad (page 91).

TARTAR SAUCE

If you're going to have a book with a recipe for crabby cakes, you must have the sauce to go with it. This tartar sauce is the perfect addition to any fried dish—it will give you the fresh taste of the sea.

MAKES ABOUT 1 CUP OF SAUCE

1 cup vegan mayonnaise
1 tablespoon whole-grain mustard
2 tablespoons sweet relish
1 teaspoon pickle juice
1 tablespoon minced red onion
1 tablespoon freshly squeezed lemon juice

1. Mix the vegan mayonnaise, mustard sweet relish, pickle juice, onion, and lemon juice together in a small bowl.

2. Place the sauce in a glass jar and store it in the refrigerator for up to 6 days.

 Perfect for Crabby Heart Cakes (page 128) or even Southern Fried Buttermilk Tofu (page 145)!

BASIL PESTO AIOLI

When I first moved to Baltimore, I would go to a sandwich shop all the time that had the most delicious basil pesto mayo. It was so simple, yet so addicting. I would get a chicken basil pesto mayo sandwich, just for this mayo spread. This was clearly before I became vegan. I don't have those chicken sandwiches anymore, but the feeling I get eating this fresh vegan version of the spread is the same.

MAKES ABOUT 1 CUP OF AIOLI

1 cup vegan mayonnaise
3 tablespoons pine nuts
½ cup chopped fresh basil
½ tablespoon garlic powder
½ teaspoon kosher salt

1. Mix the vegan mayonnaise, pine nuts, basil, garlic powder, and kosher salt in a small bowl.

2. Serve the aioli right away or store it in an airtight container in the refrigerator for up to 5 days.

 Basil Pesto Aioli is one of my favorite sandwich add-ons. It goes great with almost every savory sandwich, especially grilled vegetables!

SWEET MUSTARD DIPPING SAUCE

Growing up, my favorite meal was chicken fingers and honey mustard sauce. I was never really a picky eater, unless it came to my beloved honey mustard sauce. Like a lot of comforting meals I ate growing up, the proteins may have changed, but the flavors in my sauces certainly haven't. There's no need to give up a sweet and tangy mustard sauce even if you don't use eggs or honey. The kid in me gets excited just reading this recipe.

**MAKES 5 SERVINGS OR
ABOUT ½ CUP OF DIPPING SAUCE**

½ cup vegan mayonnaise, plus more as needed
3 tablespoons agave nectar
2 tablespoons Dijon mustard
⅛ teaspoon cayenne pepper
2 teaspoons freshly squeezed lemon juice
½ teaspoon freshly squeezed orange juice

1. Whisk the vegan mayonnaise, agave, mustard, cayenne, lemon juice, and orange juice in a small bowl.

2. If the dip is too thin, just add more vegan mayonnaise to make it your preferred consistency.

N This is the perfect dipping sauce for Fried Eggplant Sticks (page 79) or as a ketchup replacement for any veggie burger! I don't recommend just drinking it, but you'll want to.

TZATZIKI SAUCE

You're probably thinking *Cashews in tzatziki sauce?*—especially if you're new to a plant-based diet. Rest assured, you will come to learn and love that soaked cashews can make some of the thickest and creamiest sauces around. Try experimenting and come up with your own cashew-based sauce as well. This goes perfectly with a vegetable gyro or as a dipping sauce for fresh vegetables.

MAKES 4 SERVINGS OR 1⅓ CUPS OF SAUCE

1 cup raw cashews, soaked in water overnight
¼ cup water
2 tablespoons olive oil
2 tablespoons tahini
Freshly squeezed juice of ½ lemon
¼ cup minced cucumber
1 tablespoon chopped fresh dill
4 or 5 mint leaves, chopped
2 cloves garlic, minced
1 teaspoon sea salt
½ teaspoon freshly ground black pepper

1. Drain and rinse the soaked cashews.

2. In a blender, blend the cashews, water, olive oil, tahini, lemon juice, and cucumber until smooth.

3. Add the dill, mint, garlic, sea salt, and pepper and pulse until combined.

4. Serve right away or store in an airtight container in the refrigerator for up to 5 days.

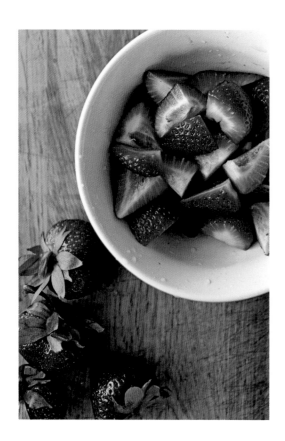

STRAWBERRY BASIL VINAIGRETTE

Tired of using salad dressings made with more ingredients that you can't pronounce than those you can? Yeah, me, too. Especially vinaigrettes. I wanted a tart yet sweet dressing without all the unnecessary chemicals. And here it is! This is my go-to dressing for all spinach- and arugula-based salads.

MAKES 2 SERVINGS OR ½ CUP OF VINAIGRETTE

1 cup fresh strawberries, chopped
3 tablespoons freshly squeezed lemon juice
2 tablespoons organic agave nectar
¼ cup extra-virgin olive oil, plus more as needed
1 tablespoon organic apple cider vinegar
3 tablespoons chopped fresh basil

1. Place the strawberries, lemon juice, agave, olive oil, apple cider vinegar, and basil in the bowl of a food processor and puree.

2. Add more olive oil if you'd like it a little thinner.

3. Put the dressing in a easy-pour container and refrigerate.

 You can store this dressing in the refrigerator for up to 14 days, but I doubt it will make it that far.

AUTUMN GLAZE

This recipe may look basic, but don't be fooled by its simplicity—it has been my go-to for almost all breakfast pastries since I started cooking. These days when I make a pastry, I use the least possible amount of sugar in the pastry itself so that I can load it up with this sweet Autumn Glaze. The sage in this glaze brings a unique freshness to your buttery pastry.

MAKES 2 SERVINGS OR ⅓ CUP OF GLAZE

¼ cup water
½ cup organic confectioners' sugar
1 teaspoon ground cinnamon
½ teaspoon freshly ground nutmeg
1 teaspoon minced fresh sage

1. Bring the water to a boil over high heat in a nonstick skillet.

2. Add the confectioners' sugar, cinnamon, and nutmeg and stir continuously until the sugar is dissolved.

3. Once the glaze has the consistency of syrup, remove it from the heat.

4. Sprinkle in the sage, mix, and let cool for 3 minutes. Use immediately.

This sweet and savory glaze goes great over all root vegetables and spice pastries.

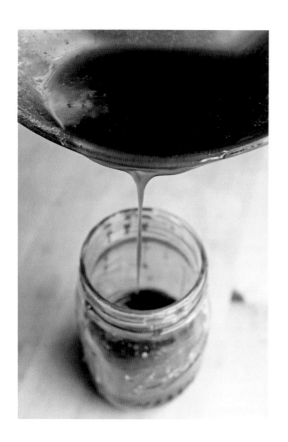

SEA-SALTED CARAMEL SAUCE

"Oh crap, I burned the caramel" is something that was once said quite a bit in my kitchen—more than I'd like to admit. But happily, my mistakes turned into this foolproof recipe, which I now offer to you. Because it uses no refined sugars, it is very forgiving (read: hard to burn!). But most important, it is absolutely delicious.

MAKES 4 SERVINGS OR ABOUT 1 CUP OF SAUCE

4 cups unsweetened organic apple juice
½ cup canned coconut milk
1 teaspoon freshly squeezed lemon juice
1 teaspoon pink Himalayan sea salt

1. Heat a medium saucepan over high heat.

2. Pour the apple juice into the hot saucepan and bring it to a boil.

3. Continue boiling until the apple juice has reduced to about 1 cup, 10 to 12 minutes.

4. Whisk the coconut milk, lemon juice, and Himalayan sea salt into the apple juice reduction until they are well combined. Then remove the pan from the heat.

5. Let the sauce cool for about 5 minutes, then transfer it to a heat-safe container and continue cooling to room temperature. Use immediately or keep in the refrigerator for up to 5 days.

COCONUT MILK CHOCOLATE SAUCE

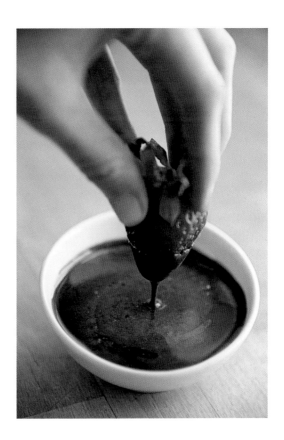

For the first year that I became vegan, I thought my only chocolate option was dark chocolate. I decided to make my own milk chocolate sauce. There was no reason I had to give up my "milk" chocolate addiction, and you don't have to either.

What to use this sauce on? Think of all the possibilities! Strawberries, pound cake, ice cream, or bananas. It's perfect no matter if you're hosting a classy dessert fondue party or if you're just lounging in your underwear on a Monday night.

MAKES A LITTLE MORE THAN 1½ CUPS OF SAUCE

1 cup coconut milk
2 tablespoons vegan butter
1½ cups semisweet chocolate chips
1 teaspoon pure vanilla extract

1. In a small saucepan, bring the coconut milk and vegan butter to a boil over medium heat.

2. Immediately remove the pan from the heat and pour in the chocolate chips. Mix until the chocolate is smooth.

3. Add the vanilla and set aside at room temperature for 30 minutes. Use immediately, or store in an airtight container in the refrigerator for up to 5 days.

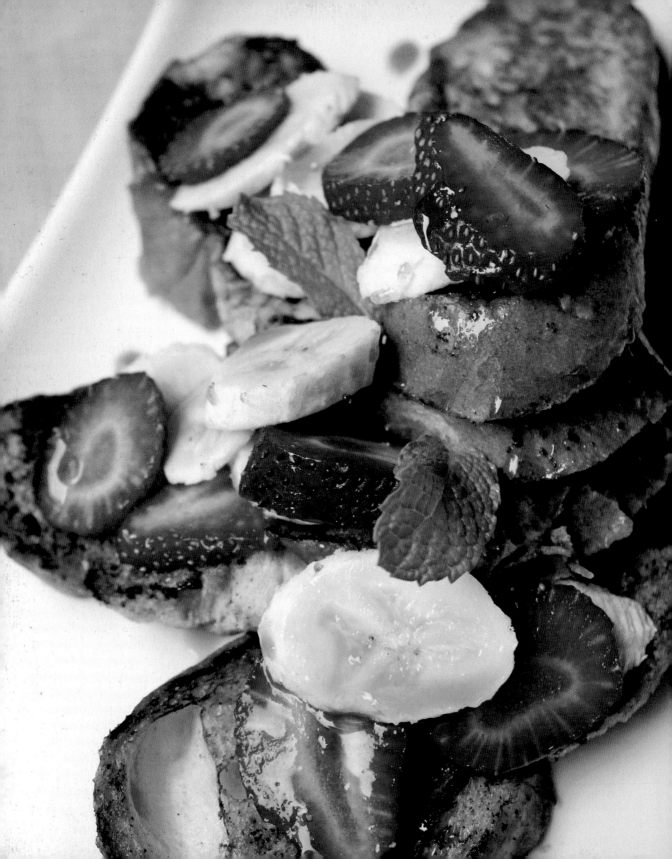

BREAKFAST

Oh, breakfast. How I hate to love thee. Breakfast is the most important meal of the day, but why does it have to be so early? For busy mornings, I recommend green smoothies for breakfast because they give you the nutrients and energy that you need for whatever task your day has in store, and green smoothies couldn't be simpler to make—just throw in some spinach, kale, hemp powder, chia seeds, banana, dates, almond milk, and ice and blend until smooth.

When you have more time or you want to indulge, though, there is a way! Scratch that—there are so many ways. Being vegan doesn't mean giving up all the traditional foods you enjoyed with your family growing up, and a good hearty breakfast is no exception. In this chapter you'll find everything from sweet to savory. These recipes are my favorite breakfast go-tos when it's just not a smoothie day. And trust me, we all have those days. So, rise and shine! Today is wonderful and your first meal awaits you. . . .

CLASSIC PANCAKES

The trick to making the perfect pancake is to use a measuring cup as your vessel to pour the batter into your skillet so that you use a consistent amount. And always, always make sure the temperature is 375 degrees F. Take a drop of water and drop it on your pan or griddle. If the water just sits there, the surface is too cold. If the water evaporates instantly, the surface is too hot. The water should essentially "dance," meaning it will move on the pan without evaporating right away!

MAKES 5 SERVINGS OR ABOUT 10 PANCAKES

2 cups sifted unbleached all-purpose flour
2 tablespoons organic granulated sugar
1 tablespoon baking powder
½ teaspoon baking soda
2 teaspoons ground cinnamon
1 teaspoon sea salt
¼ cup vegetable shortening
2 cups almond milk
1 teaspoon pure vanilla extract
Cooking spray to grease the skillet or griddle, if
   necessary

 Add chocolate chips, blueberries, or bananas to the batter if you're feeling adventurous. To be even bolder, add chives and garlic powder for some savory pancakes.

1. In a large bowl, mix the flour, sugar, baking powder, baking soda, cinnamon, and sea salt.

2. In a small bowl, mix the vegetable shortening, almond milk, and vanilla until smooth (some small chunks of shortening are okay).

3. Pour the wet ingredients into the dry ingredients and mix until well combined.

4. Heat a nonstick skillet or griddle over medium-high heat. If you don't have a nonstick skillet or griddle, then grease your pan with cooking spray.

5. Pour as much batter as you can into a measuring cup with a handle for easy pouring.

6. Pour about ¼ cup of batter for each pancake. Or go as little or as big as you'd like!

7. Once the pancakes start to bubble, 2 to 3 minutes, flip them over and cook on the opposite side for another minute or until golden brown.

8. Remove the pancakes from the pan and place them on a plate in the microwave (with the microwave off) to keep warm.

9. Repeat the process until the remaining batter is gone.

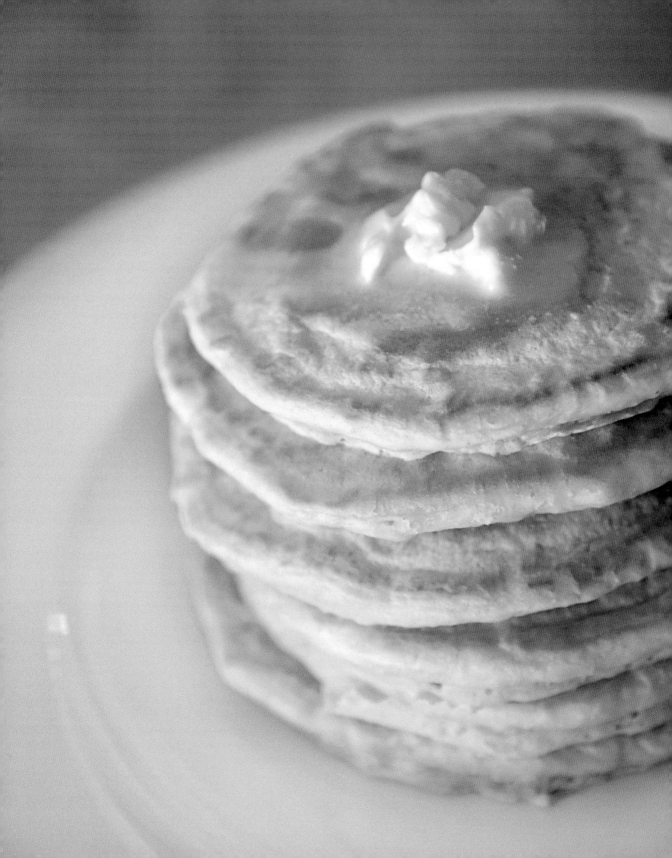

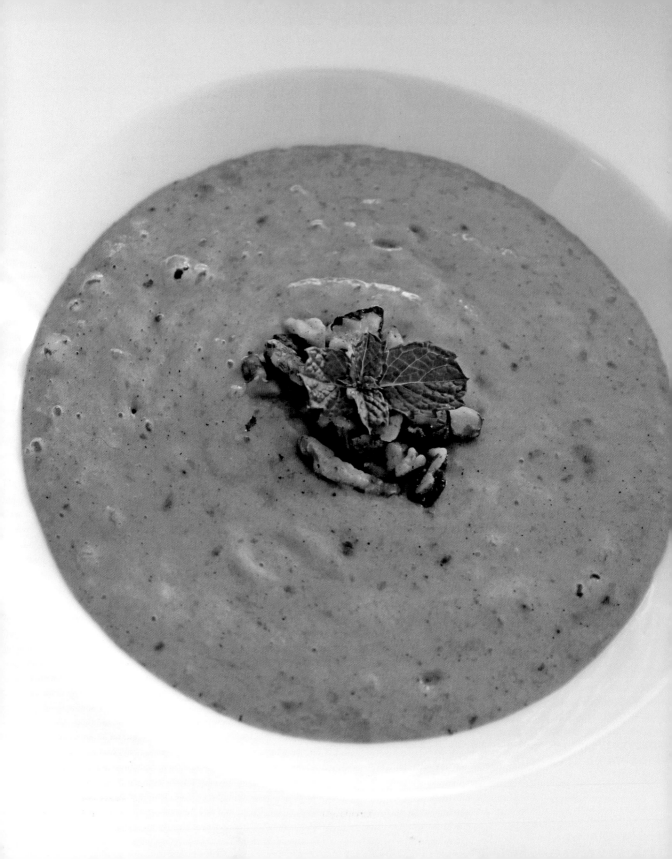

SWEET BANANA PORRIDGE

When "they" say breakfast is the most important meal of the day, "they" are right. Your body craves nutrients from the hours you've slept the night before. And you require it for fuel. If you're looking for a quick breakfast that will get you through the morning, Sweet Banana Porridge is for you. Contrary to the name, there are no actual oats in this recipe. Instead, it is an easy, fast, raw, gluten-free version of the hot cereal we all know and love. Hearty and packed with those must-have nutrients, just like a classic bowl of oatmeal, it will keep your energy up all day.

MAKES 2 CUPS OF PORRIDGE

5 ripe bananas
½ cup unsweetened almond milk
5 dates, pitted
1 teaspoon ground cinnamon
½ cup walnuts, crushed
4 mint leaves, for garnish

1. Add the bananas, almond milk, dates, and cinnamon to a blender and blend on high until smooth.

2. Place the mixture in a bowl and top with walnuts. Garnish with mint.

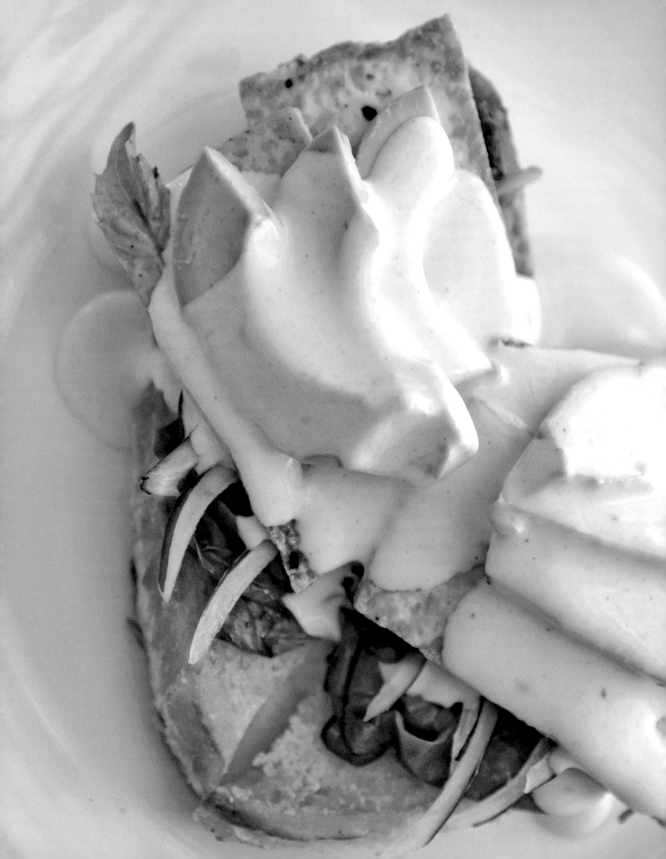

CALIFORNIA TOFU BENEDICT

Eggs Benedict was once my go-to brunch. I loved to get together with friends and make a plethora of different Benedict creations and drink mimosas. So naturally this was the first breakfast I was hell-bent on making vegan. After numerous tries, the hollandaise is just as I remember it to be. Don't be overwhelmed by a Benedict; the vegan version is actually much easier to make than its dairy and egg counterpart.

MAKES 4 SERVINGS

TOFU
1 (8-ounce) package organic extra-firm tofu, drained
1 tablespoon avocado oil
1 teaspoon garlic powder
½ teaspoon sea salt
¼ teaspoon freshly ground black pepper

HOLLANDAISE
¼ cup vegan mayonnaise
1 tablespoon water
1 teaspoon ground turmeric
¼ teaspoon kosher salt
½ teaspoon cayenne pepper
¼ teaspoon organic granulated sugar
1 tablespoon vegan butter

2 English muffins, sliced and toasted
1 cup kale, massaged
1 small avocado, pitted, peeled, and sliced
1 tomato, sliced thin
1 teaspoon chopped fresh chives
Red onion, sliced, for garnish

1. To make the totu: Preheat the oven to 350 degrees F.

2. Cut the tofu into quarters lengthwise.

3. With a circular cookie cutter, carefully cut out 4 circles from each piece of tofu. Discard the extra tofu or save for a tofu scramble the next morning.

4. In a small bowl, mix together the avocado oil, garlic powder, sea salt, and black pepper.

5. Place the tofu circles on a cookie tray lined with parchment paper and put in the oven. Bake for 20 minutes.

6. While the tofu is baking, start on the hollandaise sauce.

7. To make the hollandaise: In a small saucepan, heat the vegan mayonnaise, water, turmeric, salt, cayenne, sugar, and vegan butter over medium heat. Mix until smooth, stirring occasionally.

8. Cook for about 5 minutes, then remove from the heat and let it sit until the tofu is done.

9. Place 2 English muffins, nook-and-cranny-side up on a plate. Then place the kale, avocado, tomato, and tofu circles on top.

10. Pour the hollandaise sauce over the top of the tofu. Sprinkle with chives and enjoy!

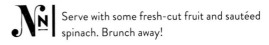 Serve with some fresh-cut fruit and sautéed spinach. Brunch away!

CRÈME DE LA CREPES

I was tempted to name this dish "I Don't Give a Crepe!" but decided against it, as that doesn't sound like the most appetizing dish. Yet the name would have been more fitting. When I stumbled upon this recipe, I was trying to make thin pancakes and accidentally made crepes instead. In the end, I couldn't have been more excited about my mistake. Don't fret if the first crepe you make breaks—it takes a bit of practice to get the flip right. My mantra in the kitchen is always to cook with care and speed, but that's especially true when it comes to crepes.

**MAKES 6 LARGE CREPES
(OR 8, IF YOU DON'T MESS UP
THE FIRST TWO LIKE I DO)**

½ cup unsweetened almond milk
½ cup water
2 tablespoons organic apple cider vinegar
¼ cup vegan margarine
1 tablespoon organic granulated sugar
1 cup sifted unbleached all-purpose flour
¼ teaspoon kosher salt
½ cup canned coconut milk, refrigerated
1 teaspoon ground cinnamon
2 tablespoons organic confectioners' sugar
1 cup fresh strawberries, stemmed and chopped
Fresh mint, for garnish

 The flipping of the crepe can be a bit tricky. I recommend using two metal spatulas to have support on both ends of the crepe. To turn these into savory crepes, simply omit the granulated sugar from the batter.

1. In a large bowl, combine the almond milk, water, apple cider vinegar, vegan margarine, granulated sugar, flour, and kosher salt.

2. Cover the bowl and let the batter chill in the fridge for 2 hours or overnight.

3. Lightly grease a nonstick skillet with some vegan margarine and heat over medium heat.

4. Pour the batter into the skillet until the bottom of the pan is lightly coated; use about 3 tablespoons of batter.

5. Swirl the pan in a circular motion to make sure the skillet is coated evenly with batter.

6. Cook until golden brown, then flip and cook the opposite side, about 1½ minutes per side. The flip side will take less time to brown.

7. Place the cooked crepe on a plate lined with a paper towel and repeat steps 4 to 6 until the batter is gone.

8. In a small bowl, fold together the coconut milk, cinnamon, and confectioners' sugar.

9. Pour the coconut mixture down the center of each crepe and top with strawberries. Then fold the crepe in from two sides toward the center, or simply fold in half.

10. Top with Coconut Milk Chocolate Sauce (page 35) and garnish with mint.

THE GLUCKY WAFFLES

One morning while I was touring with Ellie Goulding somewhere in the United States, I tried to make her assistant, Lauren Glucksman, a waffle for breakfast. Let's just say it went horribly wrong. The iron wasn't hot enough, and the batter was so stuck that I actually had to pry it off with a fork. Nonetheless, I promised I would make it up to her by perfecting a great waffle recipe she'd love and naming it in her honor. She is the queen of Peanut Butter and Jelly, so that's how The Glucky Waffles came to be. I use almond butter in this recipe because a lot of commercially made peanut butters can be high in saturated fats, salt, and sugar. Almond butter is less likely to contain those ingredients. As it gains popularity, though, be sure to always check the label and go with the product with the least number of ingredients. When picking a jam, go with whatever flavor you like best. The reason I do not use jelly is because it is almost always not vegan. It contains gelatin, which is the collagen from various animals. Stick with jam, as it tends to have fewer additives as well!

MAKES 4 HUGE WAFFLES, OR 3 CUPS OF BATTER

1½ cups gluten-free all-purpose flour
1½ teaspoons baking powder
½ teaspoon baking soda
½ teaspoon salt
1 tablespoon ground cinnamon
¼ cup (packed) organic brown sugar
1 cup unsweetened almond milk
1 tablespoon organic apple cider vinegar
½ cup water
1 teaspoon pure vanilla extract
1 tablespoon vegan butter
2 tablespoons almond butter
½ cup grape jam, or the flavor of your choosing
Cooking spray, to grease the waffle iron

1. Preheat the waffle iron so that it's ready when you're done mixing the batter.

2. In a large bowl, mix the flour, baking powder, baking soda, salt, and cinnamon.

3. In a medium bowl, mix the brown sugar, almond milk, apple cider vinegar, water, vanilla, vegan butter, and almond butter.

4. Pour the wet mixture into the dry ingredients and stir until smooth. It's okay if there are a couple chunks of almond butter—even better to bite into!

5. Pour in the jam and lightly fold it into the mixture. You don't want to mix it too much. Incorporate it, but do not mix it.

6. Once the waffle iron is hot, spray the iron with cooking spray, then pour the waffle batter evenly on the iron until the inside is filled. Do not overfill. The batter will expand.

7. Cook for 4 to 6 minutes, or until both sides are golden brown and the waffle does not stick to the iron.

 Plate with some fresh sliced bananas and pure maple syrup. Goes great with a nice glass of freshly squeezed orange juice.

BLUEBERRY OATMEAL SQUARES

Breakfast bars seem to be a new craze nowadays, and I completely understand why. Who doesn't love sweet fresh fruit with a sugary oat topping? Save yourself the heartache of the unsatisfied feeling you get when eating a processed bar, and take some time on the weekend to make these bars and portion them out to eat throughout the week. I assure you, you will feel inspired to make all different types of breakfast bars using new fruits. The creativity this recipe sparks is half the reason I love them so much.

MAKES 12 SQUARES

2½ cups gluten-free all-purpose flour
1½ cups gluten-free oats
1 cup (packed) organic brown sugar
2 tablespoons ground cinnamon
½ teaspoon baking soda
1 cup vegan butter
¼ cup water, plus cold water as needed
2 tablespoons cornstarch
2 cups blueberries
1 cup organic granulated sugar
2 tablespoons freshly squeezed lemon juice
1 teaspoon sea salt

 You can add hemp or chia seeds to the blueberry mixture to give you more pep in your step. These are great for breakfast or as dessert with some vanilla ice cream. Don't forget to garnish with mint!

1. Preheat the oven to 350 degrees F.

2. In a medium bowl, mix ½ cup of the flour, the oats, brown sugar, cinnamon, baking soda, and ½ cup of the vegan butter. Mix until well combined, then place in the refrigerator.

3. In another medium bowl, mix the water and cornstarch until the cornstarch is dissolved.

4. Add the cornstarch mixture, blueberries, granulated sugar, and lemon juice to a small saucepan and heat over medium heat.

5. Cook the blueberries for 5 to 7 minutes, stirring frequently, until the mixture starts to form a thick sauce. Remove the pan from the heat and let the mixture cool.

6. In a small bowl, mix the remaining 2 cups flour, remaining ½ cup vegan butter, and the sea salt until it forms a crumble.

7. Add cold water by the tablespoon until the mixture forms a dough. If it's too wet, add more flour. If it's too dry, add more water.

8. Line a 9 x 13-inch pan with parchment paper and press the dough into the pan until it is flat.

9. Pour the blueberry mixture over the piecrust, and crumble the chilled oat mixture over the blueberries.

10. Bake for 20 minutes or until the oats become golden brown.

11. Let cool to room temperature, then slice.

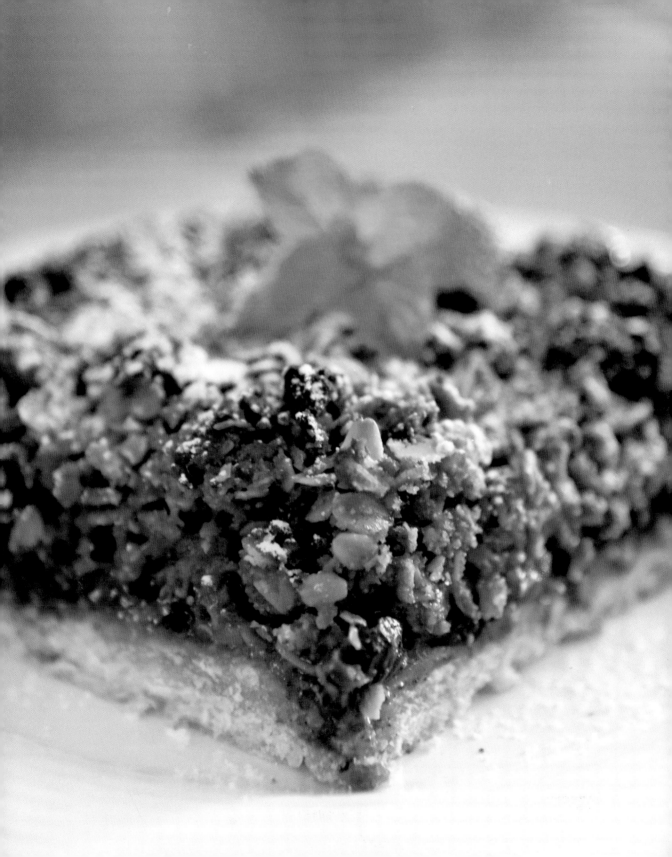

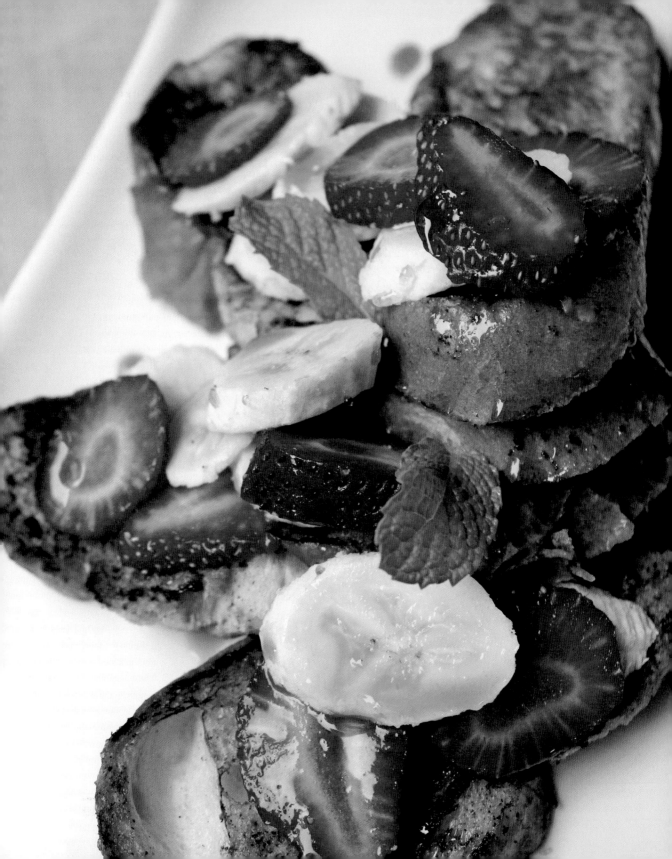

GINGERBREAD FRENCH TOAST

Growing up, the only French toast I knew of was the kind you make with presliced white bread that ends up looking like a soggy, squished version of your expectations. When I became vegan, I had the same result with every batch of French toast I made. But I've finally gotten it right. Trust me when I tell you that French toast does not need egg to be crispy on the outside and deliciously gooey on the inside. The key to the best French toast is the bread, especially when you're making a vegan version. Classic French toast is made with challah bread, which is made with egg. But not to worry—Italian bread will help you get that French toast of your dreams. Buy it unsliced from your local bakery a day before and leave the bag open overnight so it can get a bit stale. Then slice it thick to be sure the bread doesn't get too soggy. Support your local bakery *and* make the perfect French toast. Win-win.

MAKES 10 PIECES OF TOAST

2 cups nondairy milk (I prefer almond milk)
2 tablespoons sifted unbleached all-purpose flour
2 tablespoons canned coconut cream
1 tablespoon pure maple syrup
2 tablespoons ground cinnamon
1 tablespoon ground ginger
1½ teaspoons ground nutmeg
2 teaspoons pure vanilla extract
1 teaspoon sea salt
1 loaf Italian bread, unsliced
1 tablespoon vegan butter

1. In an 8 x 8-inch baking dish, mix the almond milk, flour, coconut cream, maple syrup, cinnamon, ginger, nutmeg, vanilla, and sea salt until well combined.

2. Cut the Italian bread into 1-inch-thick slices.

3. Heat a nonstick skillet over medium-high heat.

4. Melt the vegan butter in the skillet.

5. Dip the bread into the almond milk mixture until well coated. Do not saturate, just dip.

6. Place the bread in the skillet. Let the bread cook without moving it for 3 to 4 minutes, until the bottom is golden brown. Flip the bread and cook for 3 to 4 minutes more.

HEMP BANANA BERRY MUFFINS

I'm a huge fan of sneaking healthy ingredients into recipes whenever I can, especially when I can't taste them. These Hemp Banana Berry Muffins do just that. Hemp can help improve your digestive system regularity, reduces the risk of cardiovascular disease, and has been found to lower blood pressure. These muffins are perfect to make before everyone wakes up on a Saturday morning, bring to a picnic, or just eat by yourself, which is exactly what I do. They never make it out of my house, and I am completely okay with that.

MAKES 12 MUFFINS

5 tablespoons vegan margarine, at room
  temperature, plus more for greasing the muffin tin
2 cups sifted unbleached all-purpose flour
1½ teaspoons baking powder
1 teaspoon ground cinnamon
3 tablespoons hemp seeds
½ teaspoon kosher salt
¾ cup (packed) organic light brown sugar
½ teaspoon freshly squeezed lemon juice
1 cup almond milk
2 tablespoons warm water
1 banana, peeled and diced
1 cup fresh raspberries, halved

1. Preheat the oven to 350 degrees F.

2. Grease 12 cups in a muffin tin with vegan margarine.

3. In a large bowl, whisk together the flour, baking powder, cinnamon, hemp seeds, and salt.

4. Add the vegan margarine, brown sugar, lemon juice, almond milk, and warm water. Stir until the flour is no longer dry.

5. Fold in the banana and raspberries.

6. Pour the batter into each muffin cup to fill them about three-quarters of the way.

7. Bake for 30 minutes or until a toothpick inserted into the center of a muffin comes out clean.

 Add a little Autumn Glaze (page 33) on top, plus fresh strawberries and fresh mint.

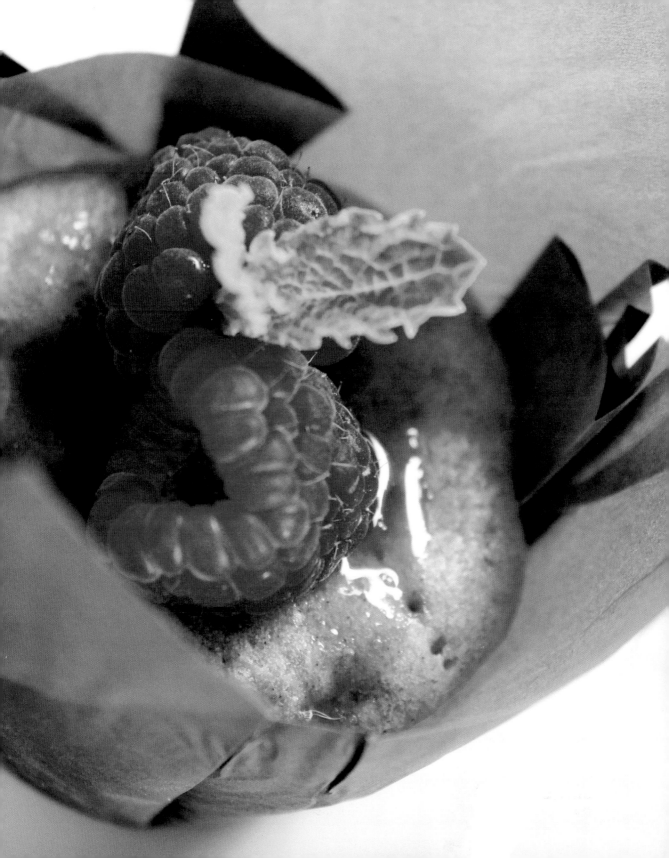

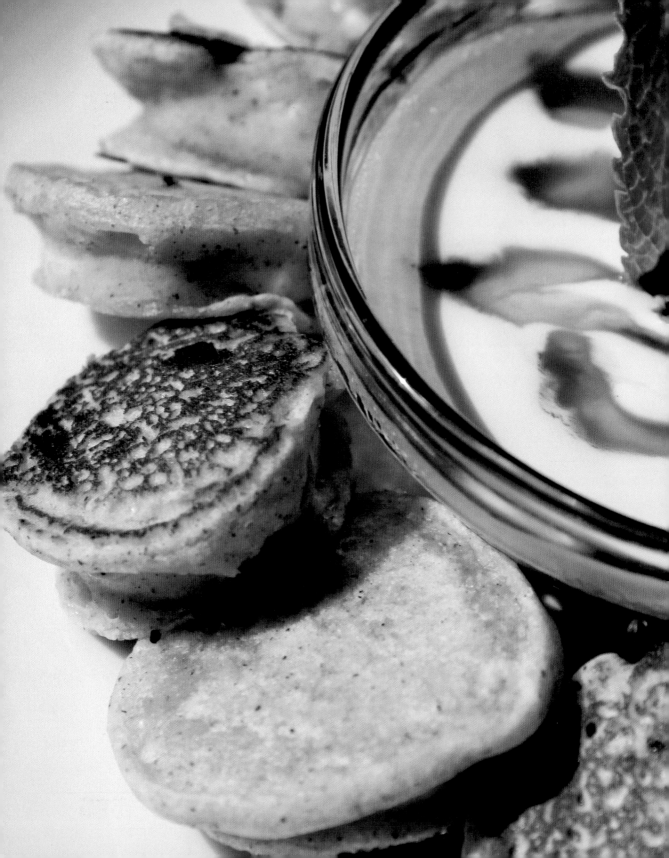

SNICKERDOODLE BANANA BITES

The marriage of bananas and pancakes is one for the ages. They are clearly meant to be together. But for a while I kept running into the same problem when I made vegan banana pancakes—the pancakes always came out way too mushy. So I created little baby versions. Because you're using such little batter for every banana bite, the batter forms a very crispy outside layer and the banana becomes creamy on the inside. To be honest, I also created this recipe because I just really want to make all of my food crispy on the outside and creamy on the inside. The process of making these bites is perfect for kiddos. However, things can get messy with this recipe. Get an apron on and get ready to embrace the sticky finger mess you are about to endure. It's worth it. If you're not into the mess (which is half the fun), then you can use a fork to dip the bananas into the batter and place them on the skillet.

MAKES 40 BANANA BITES

4 bananas, peeled
1½ cups sifted unbleached all-purpose flour
1½ tablespoons organic turbinado sugar
1 tablespoon baking powder
½ teaspoon sea salt
2 tablespoons ground cinnamon
1½ teaspoons organic apple cider vinegar
¾ cup unsweetened almond milk
½ cup water
2 tablespoons vegetable oil
2 teaspoons pure vanilla extract

1. Cut the bananas crosswise into ¼-inch slices.

2. In a medium bowl, mix the flour, turbinado sugar, baking powder, sea salt, and cinnamon.

3. Add the apple cider vinegar, almond milk, water, vegetable oil, and vanilla. Mix until smooth.

4. Heat a nonstick skillet over medium-high heat.

5. With your fingers, dip the banana slices into the batter and place them in the skillet. Cook them for about 2 minutes on each side, until golden brown.

BREAKFAST BRUSCHETTA

I was sitting at a salon and an older lady sitting next to me said, "So, what do you do?" I proceeded to tell her that I like to cook. Mind you, I had only been trying to cook for about two months at that point. She turned to me and said, "How do you pronounce that dish with tomatoes, garlic, onion, and basil?" Immediately I said, "Bruschetta?" She said, "No. Bruscketta! And you should only eat it for breakfast!" So this recipe is for that lady. I'll always remember her schooling me in the ways of bruschetta.

MAKES ABOUT 20 CROSTINIS

1 loaf French baguette
1 (8-ounce) package organic extra-firm tofu
2 tablespoons extra-virgin olive oil
2 cloves garlic, minced
½ large red onion, diced
1 cup washed and chopped baby bella mushrooms
2 cups fresh spinach
3 Roma tomatoes, diced

N If you don't have a tofu press, do not fret! There are many ways for you to get the same results. Place the tofu, wrapped in paper towels, in a deep baking dish. Place a pie pan over the tofu and place heavy food cans (or whatever heavy items you have lying around the kitchen) on top of the pie pan, and there you go! You've got yourself a makeshift tofu press!

1. Preheat the oven to 400 degrees F.

2. Using a serrated knife, cut the baguette crosswise into ¼-inch-thick slices. Get rid of the ends and save them for homemade bread crumbs!

3. Press the tofu for 30 minutes to 1 hour (see Nom Note).

4. Brush the baguette slices with some of the olive oil and place them on an 18 x 14-inch baking sheet. Bake for 5 to 6 minutes, or until golden brown. Keep an eye on them because they will burn quickly.

5. Place the rest of the olive oil, about 1 tablespoon, in a large skillet and heat over medium-high heat.

6. Place the garlic, onion, and mushrooms in the skillet and sauté for about 5 minutes, or until the garlic becomes aromatic and the onion becomes translucent.

7. Crumble the tofu with your hands gently in a large bowl. You want to keep large chunks because the tofu will crumble more in the skillet.

8. Pour the tofu into the skillet with the mushroom mixture and cook for 5 to 6 minutes.

9. Add the spinach and tomatoes and cook for 2 minutes more, or until the spinach is wilted.

10. Place a tablespoon of the tofu scramble on each baguette slice and serve hot.

TRADITIONAL GLAZED DOUGHNUTS

If you follow my website at all, you know that I am a huge fan of vegan doughnuts. I try not to make them often, but I like to know that they are possible and that being vegan doesn't mean giving up my guilty pleasures. Doughnuts absolutely take some patience, but they are more than worth it. Baked doughnuts are all right, but when you're looking for the traditional doughnut taste you probably grew up enjoying, these are the ones for you. For a thicker glaze, just cut the almond milk measurement in half. Want to add some flavor? Use the juice from your favorite fruit instead of almond milk in the glaze recipe.

MAKES 1 DOZEN DOUGHNUTS

1 tablespoon fast-acting yeast
2 cups lukewarm water
2 cups sifted unbleached all-purpose flour
¼ cup organic granulated sugar
½ teaspoon kosher salt
⅔ cup canned coconut milk, at room temperature
¼ cup vegetable shortening
4 to 5 cups peanut or safflower oil, for frying

GLAZE
1½ cups organic confectioners' sugar, sifted
¼ cup almond milk
1 teaspoon pure vanilla extract

1. In a small bowl, mix the yeast with the water and set aside until the yeast is active, about 10 minutes. You'll see the yeast start to become foamy. (Make sure the water isn't too hot or it will kill the yeast.)

2. In a large bowl, mix the flour, granulated sugar, and salt.

3. Once the yeast is active, pour it into the dry ingredients with the coconut milk and vegetable shortening.

4. Mix the ingredients together until a dough forms. If the dough is too sticky, add flour by the spoonful until the sides are no longer sticking.

5. Wet a kitchen towel with warm water and place it over the bowl. Set the bowl aside and let the dough rise until it doubles in size, about 2 hours.

6. Once the dough has risen, place it on a floured surface and roll the dough out to about ⅓ inch thick.

7. Line two 9 x 13-inch baking pans with parchment paper.

8. Cut out circles with a circle cookie cutter or a wide drinking glass. Simply poke your finger through the center of the circle to make traditional doughnuts. If you want to fill the doughnuts, leave the center as is. Place the doughnuts on the lined baking pans about 1 inch apart to give each of them room to rise again. You want 6 doughnuts on each pan.

(CONTINUED)

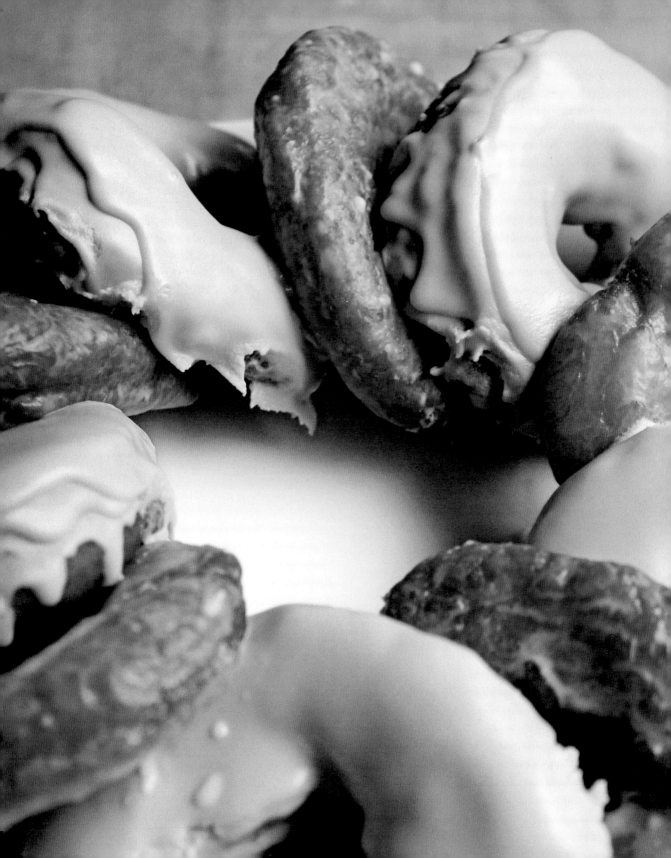

9. Place cling wrap over the doughnuts and let the doughnuts rise for another hour.

10. Heat the oil in a large pot to 375 degrees F. Use a candy/deep-fry thermometer.

11. Once the oil is ready, place each doughnut in the oil for 1 minute or until light brown, then flip to the other side using a long stick or tongs.

12. Place the fried doughnuts on a plate lined with paper towels to absorb the extra oil.

13. To make the glaze: Mix the confectioners' sugar, almond milk, and vanilla in a wide bowl and dip each doughnut in the glaze until well coated.

14. Place the doughnuts on a cooling rack with a baking sheet underneath to catch the extra glaze.

To make a vanilla cream filling for your doughnuts, blend ½ cup soaked cashew nuts, ½ cup water, ½ teaspoon pure vanilla extract, ¼ cup organic confectioners' sugar, and a pinch of coarse sea salt. Blend until smooth. To fill, place the filling in a ziplock plastic bag (or piping bag). Using scissors, cut one corner of the bag off. Once the doughnuts have cooled, use your finger to poke a hole into the side of the doughnut, until you reach the center. Place the cut-off corner of the ziplock bag into the hole and squeeze until the hole is completely filled.

TEMPEH BACON SPINACH QUICHE

Quiche without egg? you're probably thinking. Yes, quiche without egg. And let me tell you, it will fool even the pickiest of egg enthusiasts. The tempeh bacon will fool lovers of the real thing, too. This dish is the perfect savory breakfast. I like to serve it with some hash browns and fresh fruit. It makes a great meal for breakfast, lunch, or dinner!

MAKES 8 SLICES OF QUICHE

1½ cups sifted unbleached all-purpose flour or
    gluten-free flour
½ teaspoon kosher salt
1 teaspoon organic turbinado sugar
⅓ cup extra-virgin olive oil
¾ tablespoon cold water, plus more if needed
18 ounces organic extra-firm tofu
½ cup cashews, soaked and drained
1½ teaspoons garlic powder
1 teaspoon onion powder
1 teaspoon ground turmeric
½ teaspoon freshly ground black pepper
1 teaspoon sea salt
1 tablespoon coconut oil
½ medium onion, diced
1 cup chopped spinach
5 slices Maple Tempeh Bacon (page 170)
½ teaspoon smoked paprika

 Dust flour onto your pie tin before baking the quiche. It will keep the crust from sticking to the tin, without making the tin super greasy.

1. Mix the flour, kosher salt, turbinado sugar, and olive oil in a large bowl. Stir in the cold water until the dough is just combined.

2. Wrap the dough in plastic wrap and place in the freezer.

3. Preheat the oven to 350 degrees F.

4. In a blender, place the tofu, cashews, garlic powder, onion powder, turmeric, pepper, and sea salt. Blend until well combined.

5. In a medium skillet, heat the coconut oil. Add the onion and sauté until the onion is translucent. Then put the spinach on top of the onion and sauté until the spinach is wilted.

6. Chop the tempeh bacon into ¼-inch pieces.

7. Roll out the dough on a floured surface and shape it into a circle. Place it in a pie tin (see Nom Note).

8. Place half the tofu mixture in the pie tin, then pour in the spinach, onions, and tempeh bacon.

9. Cover the pie with the rest of the tofu mixture. Use a spoon to smooth out the filling and bring some of the bacon and spinach to the top.

10. Sprinkle with smoked paprika and bake for 20 minutes.

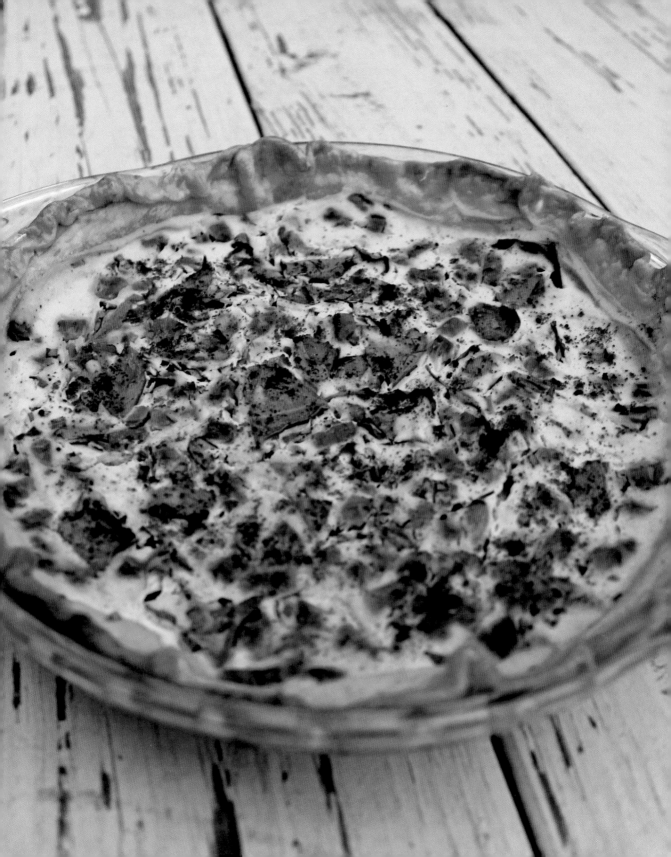

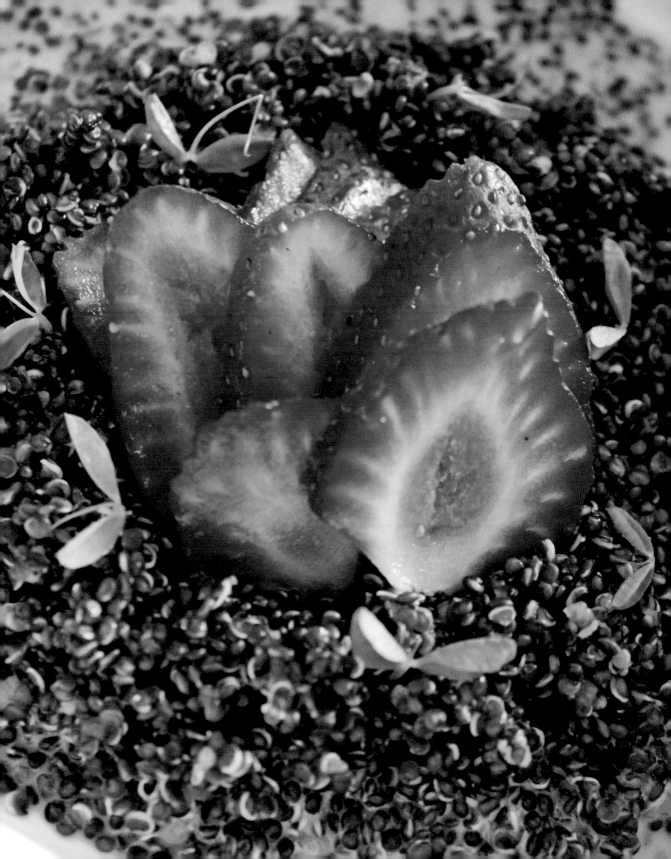

MAPLE BREAKFAST QUINOA

I have had the pleasure of cooking for actor Jeremy Piven on multiple occasions. One thing he likes is to have a filling, protein-based dish for breakfast. So I came up with a sweet quinoa that makes a great porridge with almond milk. He loved it so much the first time he tried it that the next day I showed up with a quart-size container of the stuff. You can add some nuts or granola if you'd like to give it some crunch. Quinoa is a complete protein, so it's a perfect ingredient to start your day.

**MAKES 4 SERVINGS,
OR ABOUT 2 CUPS OF QUINOA**

1 cup red quinoa
2 cups water
1 tablespoon pure maple syrup
1½ teaspoons ground cinnamon
½ teaspoon sea salt
1 cup nondairy milk

1. Rub the quinoa with your hands over a sieve under cold running water, then rinse completely. This rubbing will remove any saponins left in the outer layer of the quinoa. The saponins can have a bitter taste.

2. Place the quinoa, water, maple syrup, cinnamon, and sea salt in a large sauté pan over high heat and bring to a boil. Then reduce the heat to a simmer. Cover the pan and cook for about 15 minutes, or until all the water has been absorbed by the quinoa.

3. In a small saucepan, heat your favorite nondairy milk over high heat until it boils.

4. Once the quinoa is ready, put ½ cup of the quinoa in each of four bowls and pour ¼ cup of the nondairy milk over each serving.

5. Top with fresh fruit or granola, or eat plain!

This is a great recipe to make ahead of time. On Sunday, make several batches so you can have it for a quick breakfast throughout the week. Quinoa can be black, ivory, or red in color. I am fond of the red for its vibrant hue.

SOUTHWESTERN SCRAMBLE

Tofu scramble can be magical if it's seasoned right. I've ruined countless tofu scrambles by not adding enough spices. But the texture of the tofu is important, too. If you use watery tofu, it will end up tasting like soggy spicy tofu, so the key is to drain as much water from the tofu as possible. And use extra-firm tofu to start, especially when you make this Southwestern Scramble, because the vegetables will give off a ton of liquid as well.

MAKES 2 MEDIUM PLATES

2 tablespoons avocado oil
1 small onion, diced
3 cloves garlic, minced
1 (8-ounce) package organic extra-firm tofu
½ orange bell pepper, diced
½ red bell pepper, diced
½ cup sweet corn kernels
1 Roma tomato, diced
1 bunch of scallion, green parts only, sliced
½ teaspoon ground cumin
1 tablespoon ground turmeric
1 teaspoon sea salt
1 teaspoon freshly ground black pepper
2 ripe avocados, pulled, peeled, and chopped
¼ cup hot sauce

1. In a large, nonstick skillet, heat the avocado oil over medium heat. Add the onion and garlic and sauté until the onion is translucent.

2. Add the tofu, orange bell pepper, red bell pepper, corn, tomato, scallions, cumin, turmeric, sea salt, and black pepper to the skillet.

3. Cook for 10 minutes over medium heat.

4. Plate, then top with avocado and hot sauce.

N Have some tortillas left over? Heat them up and serve with tofu scramble for breakfast tacos.

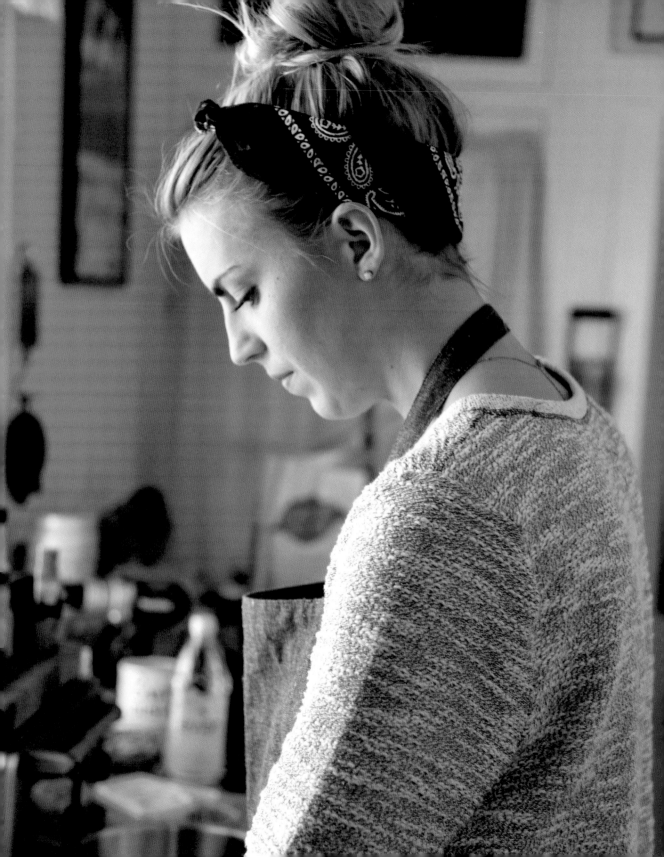

SWEET POTATO WAFFLE SANDWICH

I love sandwiches almost as much as I love anything with a crispy outside and creamy inside. I especially love breakfast sandwiches. Originally this recipe was gluten-free, which you can absolutely do by substituting gluten-free flour for the all-purpose flour, but I found the taste much better with wheat flour.

MAKES 2 FULL WAFFLES OR 4 SANDWICHES

2 tablespoons flaxseed meal
¼ cup almond milk
1 teaspoon organic apple cider vinegar
1 tablespoon coconut oil
3 cups peeled and shredded sweet potato
2 tablespoons sifted unbleached all-purpose flour
1 tablespoon chopped fresh flat-leaf parsley
1 teaspoon garlic powder
½ teaspoon freshly ground black pepper
1 teaspoon sea salt
Nonstick coconut oil spray, to grease the waffle iron
2 strips Maple Tempeh Bacon (page 170)
1 cup arugula
Hollandaise sauce (page 42)

1. In a cup or small bowl, mix together the flaxseed, almond milk, and apple cider vinegar.

2. In a large bowl, mix together the flaxseed mixture, coconut oil, shredded sweet potato, flour, parsley, garlic powder, pepper, and sea salt.

3. Heat a waffle iron and coat the waffle hot plate with nonstick coconut oil spray.

4. Pour the waffle mixture evenly on the iron until the inside is filled. Do not overfill. The batter will expand. Cook for 3 to 5 minutes or until the waffle is dark brown and crispy, depending on your waffle iron. If necessary, use a fork to help the waffle out of the waffle iron.

5. Cut each waffle in half and then in half again. Each waffle will make two sandwiches.

6. Place one waffle on a plate, top with tempeh bacon, arugula, and hollandaise sauce. Top with a second waffle. Place a toothpick in the center to hold the sandwich together.

 This may seem like a complicated breakfast sandwich, but it's really easier than it sounds, and truly one of the simpler breakfasts I make. To cut down on time, use a food processor to shred the sweet potato. The sweet potato "bun" is a great alternative for anyone who is gluten-free because you can use gluten-free all-purpose flour instead of wheat flour.

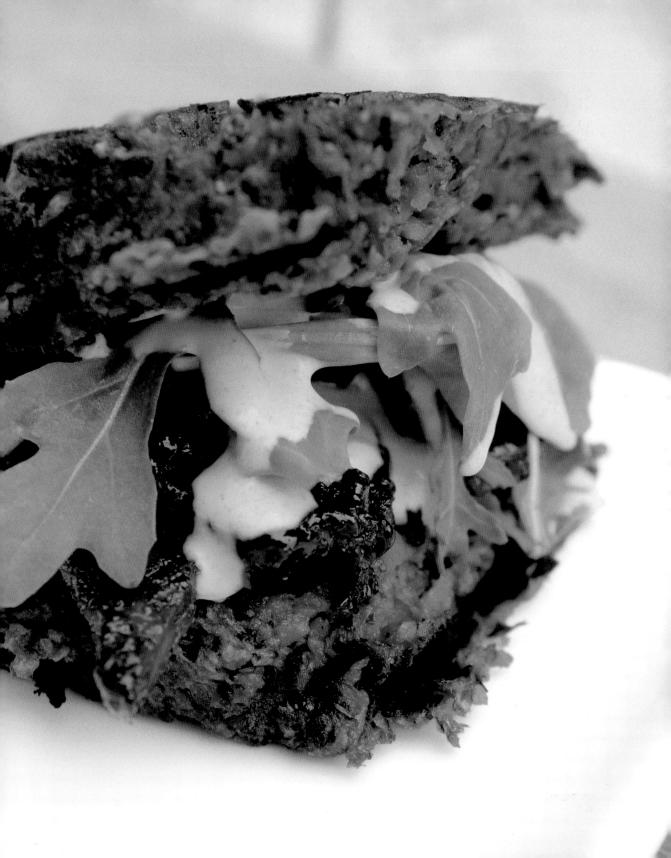

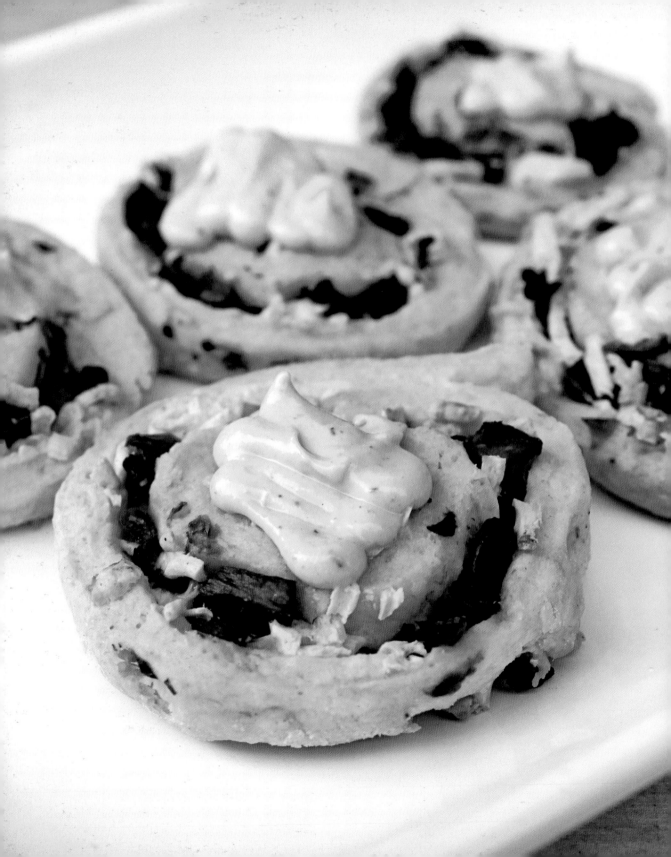

APPETIZERS

Also known as hors d'oeuvres, meaning "apart from the work," appetizers—usually small finger foods like bruschetta, canapés, crudités, dumplings, spanakopita, and much more—are the first course to any dining experience and can set the tone for the event. They are the cook's way of saying, "Get ready for what's to come." Simple and flavorful, they whet your guests' appetites and keep them happy before the main course is served.

And, confession: they're usually my favorite course! There's something I just can't resist about these "miniature meals," as I think of them. Plus, they're a great low-stakes way to get creative in the kitchen. Don't have tomatoes for bruschetta? Use sweet potatoes instead. Or cucumbers! Think outside the box. You may be surprised what you're capable of. Now go create delicious miniature pieces of art!

CANNELLINI CAPRESE CROSTINI

No time to make a nut-based cheese for your party? No problem. Cannellini beans make for an amazing savory, creamy appetizer at parties. These caprese crostini are simple and defined. No cheese necessary! I love anything you can put on toasted French bread, especially when it has the smooth, rich texture and vibrant taste of cannellini beans. Once upon a time, cannellini beans were the last beans I used from my pantry. Not anymore. If you can't find cannellini beans, don't fret. Navy beans are a perfect alternative as they are very close in taste and shape, just a little smaller in size.

MAKES ABOUT 24 CROSTINI

¼ cup vegan margarine, softened
3 teaspoons garlic powder
1 loaf French bread, cut into ½-inch slices
1 can cannellini beans, drained and rinsed
2 tablespoons freshly squeezed lemon juice
¼ cup olive oil
1 teaspoon dried oregano
¼ teaspoon sea salt
2 medium tomatoes, thinly sliced
¼ cup chopped fresh basil
¼ cup balsamic vinegar
Extra-virgin olive oil, for drizzling
Salt and freshly ground black pepper

1. Preheat the oven to 400 degrees F.

2. In a small bowl, mix together the vegan margarine and 1½ teaspoons of the garlic powder. Brush the garlic margarine on each slice of bread, then place the bread on a baking sheet.

3. Bake for 10 minutes, or until golden brown. Keep an eye on these guys; they will burn quickly.

4. In a blender, place the cannellini beans, lemon juice, olive oil, oregano, remaining 1½ teaspoons garlic powder, and the sea salt.

5. Pulse until the mixture is well combined and the beans are smooth.

6. Once the French bread is done, spread the bean mixture on top of each slice. Then top with tomatoes.

7. Sprinkle with basil and drizzle with balsamic vinegar and a touch of extra-virgin olive oil. Add salt and pepper to taste.

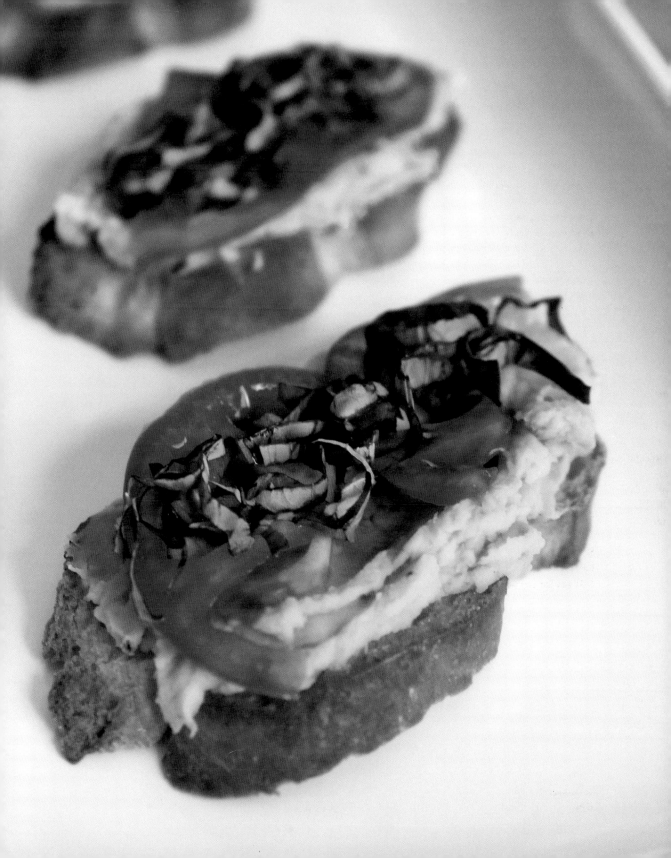

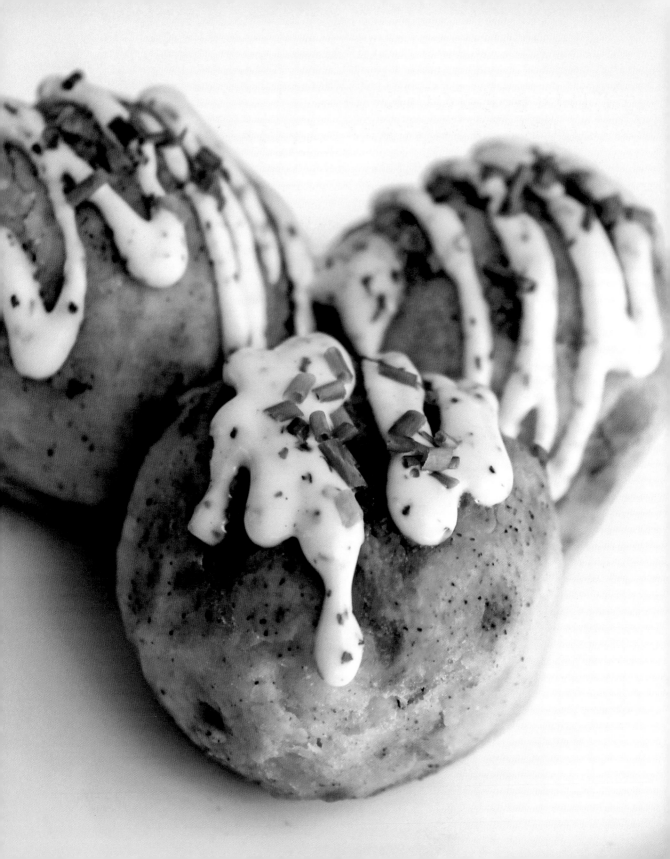

CHIVE BACON MASHED POTATO SPHERES

This recipe was inspired by my love for arancini, Italian fried rice balls stuffed with goodies. There's something magical about forming different ingredients into perfect balls, frying them, and then cracking them open as you eat. The texture of these mashed potato spheres is heavenly: crispy on the outside, soft and fluffy on the inside. They go great with my Buttermilk Ranch Dip (page 28)!

MAKES ABOUT 24 SPHERES

3 cups mashed potatoes
¼ cup vegan margarine
3 tablespoons minced fresh chives, plus more for garnish (optional)
3 strips Maple Tempeh Bacon, chopped (page 170)
1 teaspoon garlic powder
1 teaspoon sea salt
1 cup sifted unbleached all-purpose flour
1 teaspoon baking powder
1 cup almond milk
½ cup peanut oil

 You can use gluten-free flour for this recipe. To avoid that strong garbanzo bean flour taste usually found in most gluten-free all-purpose flours, just spice up your mashed potatoes by adding chili powder or hot sauce. I sometimes add a little kick even when I'm not using gluten-free flour.

1. In a large bowl, mix the mashed potatoes and vegan margarine and let stand at room temperature for 20 minutes.

2. Add the chives, tempeh bacon, garlic powder, and ½ teaspoon of the sea salt and mix.

3. Shape the mixture into 1½-inch spheres and place them on parchment paper until all the potato mixture has been used up.

4. In a medium bowl, mix together the flour, baking powder, and remaining ½ teaspoon sea salt.

5. In a separate medium bowl, put the almond milk.

6. Heat the peanut oil in a deep skillet over medium-high heat. The oil should be about 350 degrees F.

7. Roll the mashed potato spheres in the flour mixture, then milk, then the flour mixture again.

8. Place the floured spheres in the hot peanut oil and roll until they are golden brown everywhere. Do not crowd the spheres in the oil because you will need room to roll them around.

9. Place the golden brown spheres on a plate lined with paper towels to absorb some of the oil.

10. Serve with Buttermilk Ranch Dip (page 28) and top with extra chives, if desired.

GUACAMOLE WONTONS

I try to step outside of the box when it comes to using ingredients in new ways in my recipes. Avocado is one example. Yes, avocados are great just on a piece of toast. But I also love them whipped into guacamole and fried into beautiful, crispy triangles! This is a perfect recipe for when you need to feed a lot of people quickly. Just watch your oil and make sure it doesn't smoke.

**MAKES ABOUT 30 WONTONS
(IF YOU CAN KEEP FROM EATING
THE GUACAMOLE BEFOREHAND)**

2 cups peanut oil, for frying

2 ripe avocados, pitted, peeled, and cubed

2 tablespoons chopped fresh cilantro, plus more for
  garnish

½ red onion, diced

3 Roma tomatoes, minced

2 teaspoons freshly squeezed lime juice

1 clove garlic, minced

1 teaspoon sea salt

30 vegan wonton wrappers

1. Heat the peanut oil in a medium skillet over medium-high heat to 350 degrees F. Use a candy/deep-fry thermometer.

2. In a medium bowl, gently fold together the avocados, cilantro, onion, tomatoes, lime juice, garlic, and sea salt.

3. Fill a small bowl with ice water. Gently dip your finger in, then trace the outline of the wonton wrapper.

4. Fill the center of the wonton wrapper with 1½ teaspoons of the guacamole and fold over to make a triangle. Press along the edges to make sure they don't come undone.

5. Fry the wontons in the hot oil for 1 to 1½ minutes, until golden brown. Do not crowd the wontons in the skillet. Make sure you fry only 3 or 4 at a time, depending on the pan size.

6. Remove the wontons from the pan and place on paper towels to cool and to let any excess oil drip off.

7. Serve hot with Coconut Sour Cream (page 18) and fresh cilantro.

 You're going to want to double this recipe for parties. Whenever I make them, they are always the first snack gone. Make sure to save some for yourself! Having a hard time finding vegan wonton wrappers? Don't sweat it. Head to your local Asian market and you should be able to find them in the freezer section.

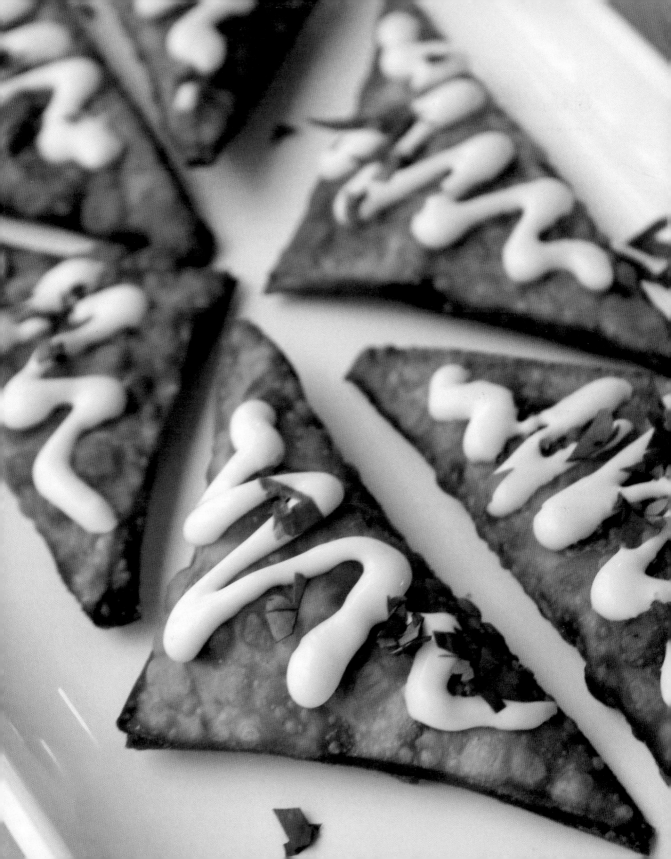

PIE WHEELS

I think there is a recipe for some sort of savory-filled wheel on the back of every prepackaged croissant or biscuit container, which is why I am so familiar with these guys. They are essentially the savory version of a frosted cinnamon roll. Pie Wheels remind me of family parties and capture the quintessential modern "make it fast" style of American cooking. My version is a bit healthier but just as easy to make. Don't have packaged vegan cheese lying around? Use Cashew Cream (page 16) instead!

MAKES ABOUT 20 WHEELS

1½ cups sifted unbleached all-purpose flour
½ teaspoon kosher salt
½ teaspoon organic granulated sugar
½ cup (1 stick) vegan margarine
4 tablespoons ice water
1 cup baby bella mushrooms, washed and diced
3 medium shallots, peeled and sliced
1 large red bell pepper, diced
1 cup vegan mozzarella cheese

1. Preheat the oven to 350 degrees F.

2. In a large bowl, combine the flour, kosher salt, and sugar. Mix until the ingredients are well combined.

3. Using a fork, cut in 6 tablespoons of the vegan margarine.

4. Add the ice water one tablespoon at a time, until the dough can form a ball. If the dough is too dry, add more ice water one tablespoon at a time.

5. Wrap the dough ball in plastic wrap and place it in the refrigerator.

6. In a medium skillet, heat the remaining 2 tablespoons vegan margarine over medium heat.

7. Add the baby bella mushrooms and shallots. Sauté for 4 to 5 minutes, until the mushrooms are a dark brown and the shallots are soft. Then set aside.

8. Take the dough out of the refrigerator and roll it out on a floured surface. Try as much as possible to shape the dough into a rectangle.

9. Spread the mushrooms and shallots across the dough, covering the surface of the dough. Sprinkle red bell pepper and vegan mozzarella on top of the mushrooms and shallots.

10. Carefully roll the dough up from one end, forming a long cylinder.

11. With a chef's knife, cut the cylinder crosswise into ¼-inch slices to form circles.

12. Place the circles, or "wheels," with the filling facing up, on a baking sheet lined with parchment paper.

13. Bake for 25 minutes or until the crust is golden brown.

You can fill the dough with whatever veggies you have lying around. Just remember to roast or sauté the diced vegetables before filling the dough with them. Mix 1 ripe avocado with Buttermilk Ranch Dip (page 28) as a topping and you've got yourself a nice little hors d'oeuvre.

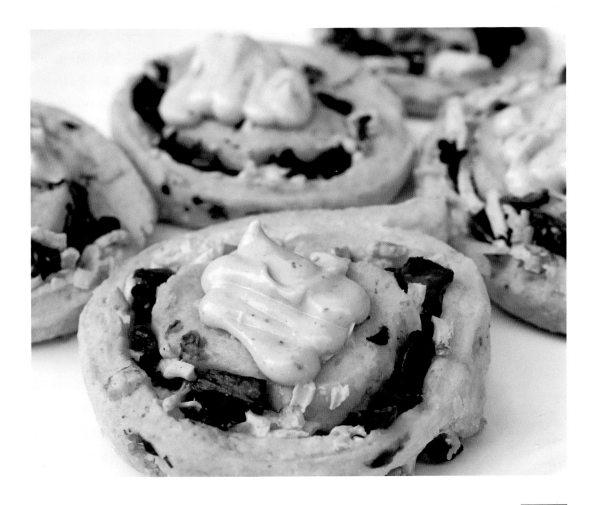

GARLIC POTATO KALE CAKES

This recipe came out of a pretty horrible kitchen experience I had. I was sautéing kale for a simple dinner of kale, mashed potatoes, and roasted vegetables. I use kitchen towels for the handles of my skillets because they generally get pretty hot, but the kitchen towel I was holding slid and my hand hit the flame on the stove. The skillet went flying and landed in the bowl of potatoes. Somehow, this event helped me come up with the idea to just pan-fry them together. Sometimes your mistakes turn into beautiful pieces of art. Hopefully you can tell by now that I love anything that's crispy on the outside and creamy on the inside. Fritters, grilled cheese, perfectly fried french fries, arancini, crabless cakes, you name it. These are on the top of the list.

MAKES 6 CAKES

6 russet potatoes, peeled, cubed, and cooked
3 cups finely chopped kale leaves
½ cup unsweetened almond milk
1 tablespoon vegan margarine
3 tablespoons sifted unbleached all-purpose flour
1 clove garlic, minced
1 teaspoon onion powder
1 tablespoon chopped fresh flat-leaf parsley
½ teaspoon freshly ground black pepper
1 teaspoon sea salt
2 tablespoons vegetable oil
1 bunch of scallions, sliced, for garnish

1. After draining the potatoes, return them to the same pot. Add the kale and toss so the heat from the potato wilts the kale leaves, about 5 minutes.

2. Once the kale is wilted, add the almond milk, vegan margarine, flour, garlic, onion powder, parsley, pepper, and sea salt.

3. Blend with an immersion blender (or blend in batches in a regular blender) until mostly smooth, with a handful of potato chunks. You want it to have some texture.

4. Heat the vegetable oil in a large skillet over medium-high heat.

5. Shape the kale-potato mixture with your hands into ¼-inch-thick patties. Place them on parchment paper.

6. Once the oil is hot, use a metal spatula to place the cakes in the oil. Cook for 2 to 3 minutes on each side, or until golden brown.

7. Transfer the patties to a plate and top each with a dollop of Buttermilk Ranch Dip (page 28) or Coconut Sour Cream (page 18) and scallion.

 Serve with roasted veggies and Cauliflower Steak (page 127) and then dare someone to tell you that they could never be vegan because they're a steak-and-potatoes kind of person.

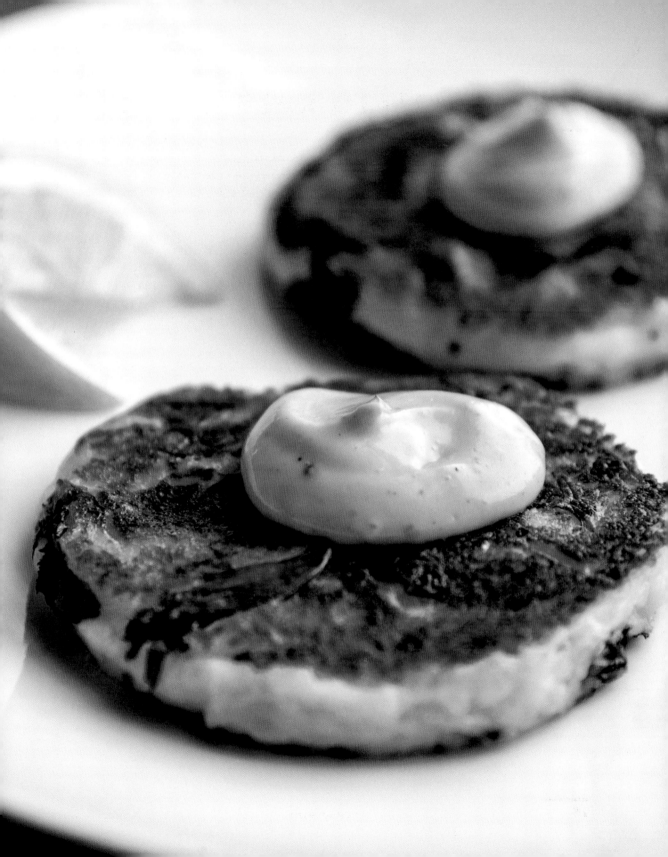

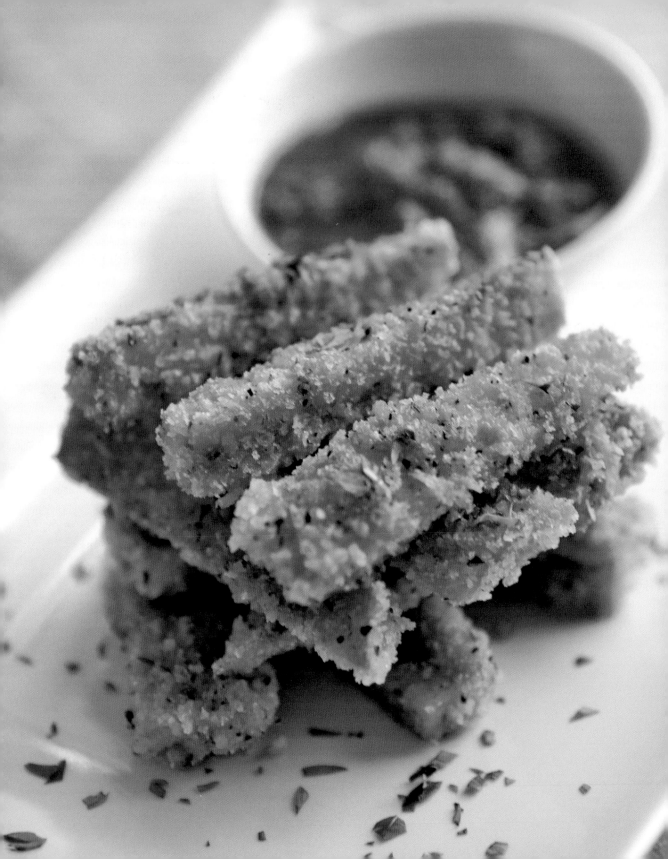

FRIED EGGPLANT STICKS

Mozzarella sticks are the ultimate crowd-pleasing appetizers. Who doesn't love a snack you can dip? My favorite vegetable has always been eggplant, and it turns out that when eggplant is breaded and fried, it makes a perfect creamy filling, even better than mozzarella. Zucchini sticks are great as well, but they tend to fall apart more often than not. So I've found that eggplant works best for an irresistible vegan twist on a favorite that everyone will want to eat by the plateful. This appetizer is by far my personal chef clients' favorite.

MAKES ABOUT 20 STICKS

1 cup sifted unbleached all-purpose flour
1 cup unsweetened almond milk
1 cup bread crumbs
1 teaspoon garlic powder
1 teaspoon onion powder
2 teaspoons finely chopped fresh flat-leaf parsley
½ teaspoon kosher salt
Peanut oil, for frying
1 large eggplant, peeled and sliced into sticks

1. Place the flour in one bowl and the almond milk in another bowl.

2. In a third bowl, mix the bread crumbs, garlic powder, onion powder, parsley, and kosher salt.

3. Place the bowls next to one another in this order: flour, almond milk, bread crumbs.

4. Add enough peanut oil to a large skillet to have the oil ½ inch deep. Heat the oil over medium heat to 350 degress F. Use a deep fry candy thermometer.

5. Dip each stick of eggplant in the flour, then the almond milk, then the bread crumbs.

6. Place the eggplant sticks in the hot oil and cook until golden brown, around 45 seconds. You may need to turn them depending on how hot your oil is.

7. Place on a plate lined with a paper towel to drain off the excess oil.

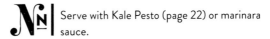 Serve with Kale Pesto (page 22) or marinara sauce.

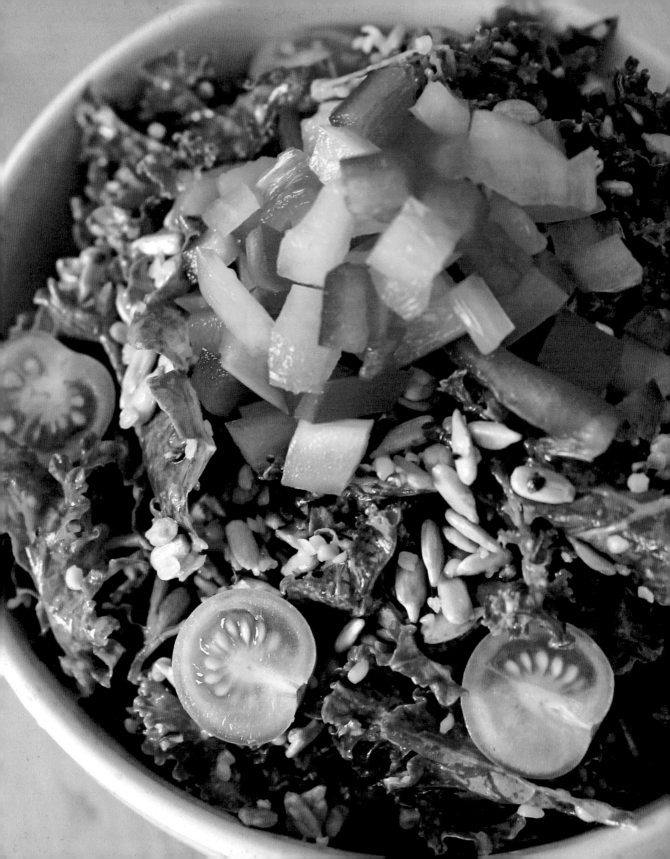

SOUPS & SALADS

Since my father became vegan, he has turned into a true soup-and-salad man, and eats a hearty soup with a light salad for dinner nearly every day. It's become his staple. At first I was skeptical, because to be honest, soups and salads used to be dishes that I'd have a few bites of while I waited for the "real" meal to come out. But watching him chow down happily on his soup-salad combo inspired me to start doing the same, and now a steaming bowl of rich soup paired with a light, fresh salad has become my go-to dinner option. For you skeptics out there who are picturing a sad bowl of greens with a tomato or two in there, with a side of soup from a can, you're in for a treat.

BLACK BEAN JAMBALAYA 82

SWEET ROASTED PUMPKIN SOUP 85

CHIPOTLE BBQ QUINOA CHILI 86

KALE NOODLE SOUP 88

SWEET SENSATION SALAD 89

BUFFALO CAULIFLOWER KALE SALAD 91

BELL PEPPER KALE SALAD 92

SUMMER SALAD 95

BLACK BEAN JAMBALAYA

For as long as I can remember I've been in love with New Orleans culture, and jambalaya is a huge part of the Creole cuisine there. For generations this traditional dish has been made with four parts: meat, vegetables, stock, and rice. I've cut out the meat and replaced it with TVP, which stands for textured vegetable protein. It has the same feel as ground beef would and absorbs any flavor you add to it. I can tell you there's still a deep, soulful flavor in this dish without the meat, and what's more, your kitchen will smell like you've brought a piece of Louisiana home with you. So turn on the jazz and get cooking!

MAKES 4 MEDIUM BOWLS

1 tablespoon vegan margarine
½ cup textured vegetable protein (TVP)
1 small red onion, minced
2 tablespoons smoked paprika
1 tablespoon ground cumin
½ teaspoon cayenne pepper
1 teaspoon dried oregano
1 teaspoon garlic powder
½ teaspoon freshly ground black pepper
1 teaspoon sea salt
1 cup diced Roma tomatoes
1 large green bell pepper, diced
2 stalks celery, diced
1 cup uncooked brown rice
4 cups Vegetable Broth (page 19)
2 cups canned black beans, rinsed
Coconut Sour Cream (page 18) (optional)
Hot sauce (optional)
2 scallions, greens and whites, chopped (optional)

1. In a Dutch oven or heavy-bottomed pot with a lid, melt the vegan margarine over medium-high heat.

2. Add the TVP and onion. Cook until the TVP has become a darker brown, about 4 minutes.

3. Add the paprika, cumin, cayenne, oregano, garlic powder, black pepper, and sea salt. Cook for 1 minute more.

4. Add the tomatoes, bell pepper, and celery. Cook, stirring, for 5 minutes more.

5. Pour in the rice and stir until well combined, then add the vegetable broth and black beans. Bring to a simmer.

6. Reduce the heat to low, cover the pot, and cook the mixture for 1 hour.

7. Remove the lid and check the rice. It should be tender. If not, cook for 5 minutes more or so.

8. Ladle the jambalaya into a bowl and serve topped with a dollop of Coconut Sour Cream, hot sauce, and scallions, onion, if desired.

 Sliced French bread serves as a great spoon for this dish!

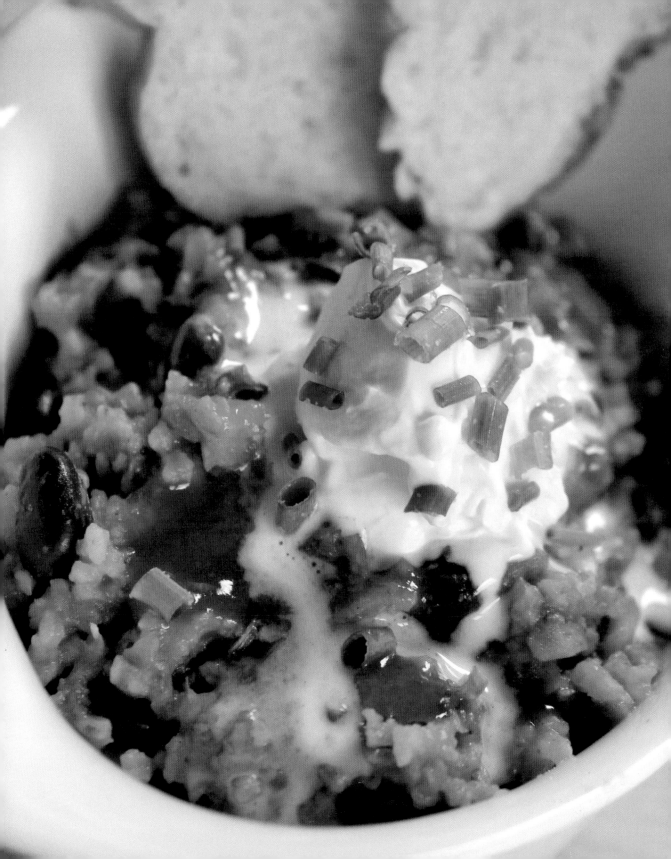

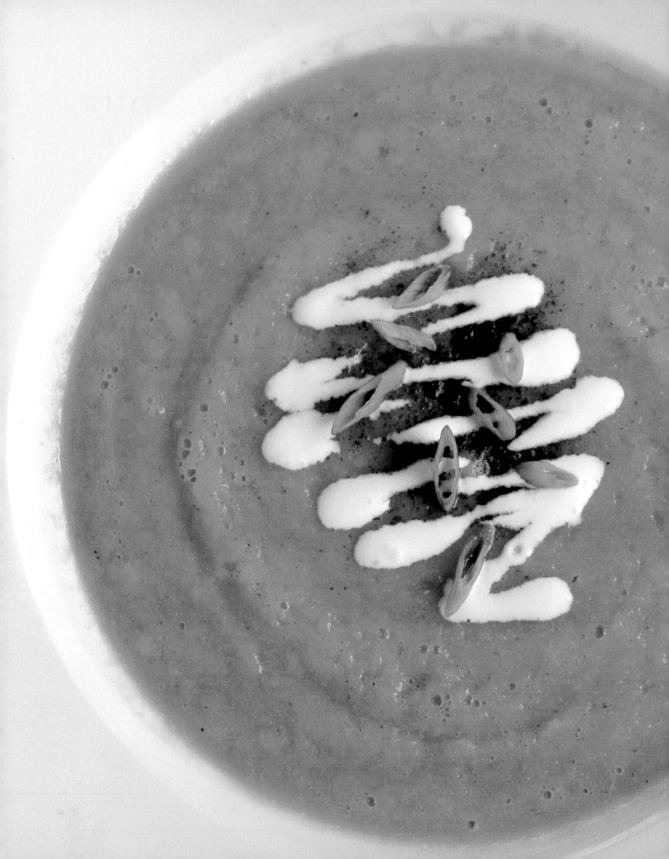

SWEET ROASTED PUMPKIN SOUP

I've never been a huge fan of plain pumpkin. It always has a bitter taste when it's just roasted, in my opinion. Most people never even really try pumpkin unless it's in the form of a pumpkin pie—which, don't get me wrong, is delicious! But you can also enjoy pumpkin in a savory soup with just a few ingredients to bring out its best qualities. So when they're in season, make sure to grab some extra at the farm for this recipe! The best pumpkin for cooking is the sugar pie pumpkin.

MAKES 5 CUPS OF SOUP

1 medium pumpkin
3 tablespoons coconut oil
1 large yellow onion, chopped
2 medium carrots
4 cups Vegetable Broth (page 19)
1 tablespoon coconut cream
2 tablespoons pure maple syrup
Dash of ground cinnamon
Sea salt to taste

1. Preheat the oven to 375 degrees F. Slice the pumpkin in half and remove the stem and seeds. Place the pumpkin halves on a baking sheet with the skin facing up.

2. Bake the pumpkin for 1½ hours.

3. Once the pumpkin is roasted and soft when poked with a fork, let cool a bit, then remove the skin.

4. In a large pot, heat the coconut oil over medium heat. Add the onion and carrots and sauté them for 5 to 6 minutes, until the carrots are soft.

5. Add the vegetable broth, coconut cream, maple syrup, cinnamon, and sea salt.

6. Cook for about 10 minutes over medium heat, or until the mixture is well heated.

7. Mash the pumpkin well so that there are just a few (or no) chunks remaining.

8. Pour the pumpkin mixture into a blender and blend until smooth. Make sure to vent the lid so that the heat isn't contained in the blender.

 Top this delicious soup with Coconut Sour Cream (page 18), cinnamon, sunflower seeds, and whatever fresh herbs you have in the house. I suggest scallions or cilantro. If pumpkins are not in season, use another squash, such as butternut or acorn squash.

CHIPOTLE BBQ QUINOA CHILI

You are either a sweet chili person or a spicy chili person. I am very much a sweet chili person. But most of the chilies I've ever had have been either extremely spicy or very bland. I created this recipe to find a happy balance of sweet flavor, without sacrificing the spicy kick because, after all, it's called chili for a reason. This dish is perfect for cold, rainy nights.

MAKES 6 MEDIUM BOWLS OF CHILI

1 tablespoon coconut oil
1 cup diced yellow onion
3 stalks celery, diced
3 cloves garlic, minced
2 tomatoes, diced
1 cup quinoa, rinsed and cooked
1 cup black beans, rinsed
1 cup kidney beans, rinsed
2 sweet potatoes, peeled and finely chopped
3 cups Vegetable Broth (page 19)
1 teaspoon liquid smoke
¼ cup ketchup
1 tablespoon chili sauce
½ cup strong coffee
3 tablespoons (packed) organic brown sugar
3 tablespoons organic apple cider vinegar
Freshly squeezed juice of ½ lemon
1 teaspoon smoked paprika
1 teaspoon ground cumin
1½ teaspoons stone-ground mustard
3 zucchini, chopped
1 carrot, shredded, for plating
1 bunch of fresh sage, chopped, for plating

1. In a large pot, heat the coconut oil over medium-high heat. Add the onion, celery, and garlic. Sauté for about 4 minutes, until the onion is soft.

2. Reduce the heat to medium and add the tomatoes, quinoa, black beans, kidney beans, sweet potatoes, vegetable broth, liquid smoke, ketchup, chili sauce, coffee, brown sugar, apple cider vinegar, lemon juice, paprika, cumin, mustard, and zucchini.

3. Cover the pot, reduce the heat to low, and simmer for 20 minutes, or until the chili has thickened.

4. Top with Coconut Sour Cream (page 18), carrot, and sage. Serve with toast and enjoy!

The great thing about chili, aside from being delicious, is that you can really put whatever you want in it. Don't like zucchini? Switch it for eggplant or add more beans. Chili does not judge. As long as you keep the measurements consistent, the world is your oyster.

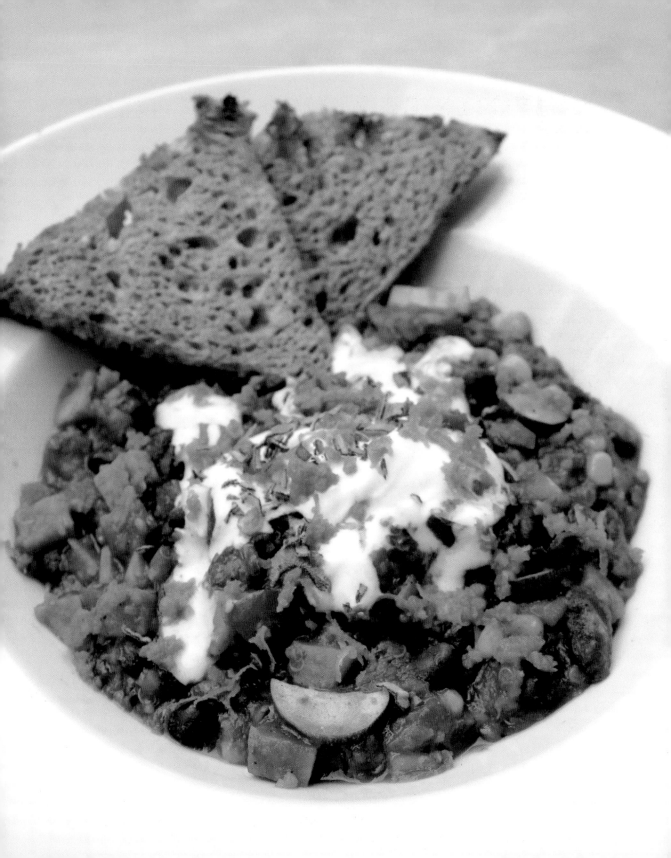

KALE NOODLE SOUP

What better way to cure a cold or sickness than with noodle soup? Most of us grew up eating chicken noodle soup, and for a lot of us it came out of a can. It's easy to make a vegan noodle soup with very simple ingredients that's much lower in sodium than store-bought canned soup. This nutritious kale noodle soup will actually help heal you. Isn't that exactly what we should be eating when we're sick?

MAKES 5 CUPS OF SOUP

3 tablespoons coconut oil
1 large yellow onion
3 cloves garlic, minced
3 large carrots, sliced
4 stalks celery, halved lengthwise and chopped
1½ cups white mushrooms, washed and chopped
2½ cups Vegetable Broth (page 19)
1½ cups water
1 teaspoon sea salt
3 cups chopped kale leaves
1 handful of lo mein noodles
1 handful of fresh flat-leaf parsley, chopped,
   for garnish

1. Heat the coconut oil in a large pot over medium-high heat.

2. Add the onion, garlic, carrots, celery, and mushrooms to the pot and sauté for 5 to 6 minutes, until the onion is tender.

3. Add the vegetable broth, water, and sea salt. Bring the mixture to a boil.

4. Add the kale. Reduce the heat and simmer for 20 minutes.

5. Add the lo mein noodles and cook for another 6 minutes.

6. Garnish with parsley and serve.

SWEET SENSATION SALAD

Before I became vegan, I ate this salad for lunch almost every day, not even realizing that it was vegan. I would make a big batch of it, then stick it in the fridge and have it for the week. It has crunch from the walnuts, saltiness from the capers, and sweetness from the cranberries—the perfect trinity of flavors for a salad. Don't let anyone tell you salads are boring!

MAKES 2 MEDIUM SALADS

2 cups baby spinach or chopped spinach
1 head of romaine lettuce, chopped
3 tablespoons capers
2 pears, peeled, cored, and thinly sliced
1 cup chopped walnuts
¼ cup dried cranberries
3 tablespoons Strawberry Basil Vinaigrette (page 32)

1. In a large bowl, mix the spinach and romaine.

2. Add the capers, pears, walnuts, and dried cranberries. Toss.

3. Place the salad in the middle of the plate with room around the edges.

4. Drizzle the dressing on the outside of the salad and serve.

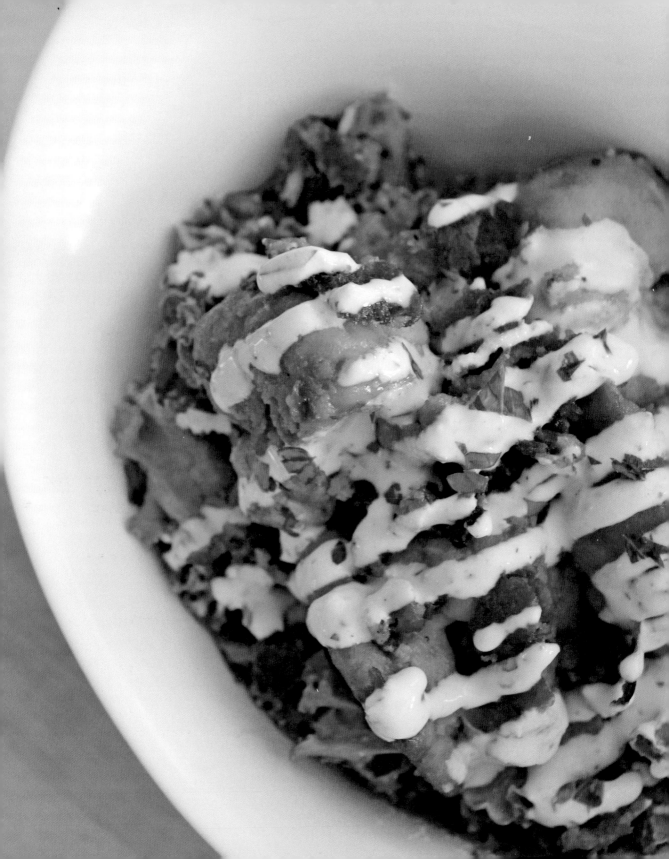

BUFFALO CAULIFLOWER KALE SALAD

One of my favorite to-go restaurants in New York City, Blossom du Jour has a kale salad entrée and a Buffalo-cauliflower bites side dish on their menu. One day I wanted a hearty salad, something more than just a mouthful of massaged kale, so I ordered both dishes and combined them, then topped it with some ranch dressing. Delicious and satisfying, it totally hit the spot. And this recipe was born! This is a salad even the biggest meat eaters can get into.

MAKES 4 SERVINGS OF SALAD

1½ cups water
¾ cup sifted unbleached all-purpose flour
1½ teaspoons garlic powder
1 teaspoon baking powder
Pinch of salt
1 medium head of cauliflower, cut into bite-size pieces
Coconut oil cooking spray
2 tablespoons coconut oil
½ cup hot sauce (I prefer Frank's RedHot)
2 cups chopped kale leaves
Buttermilk Ranch Dip (page 28)

 To take the healthy factor of this recipe to the next level, nix the batter and roast the cauliflower instead.

1. Preheat the oven to 450 degrees F.

2. Mix the water, flour, garlic powder, baking powder, and salt in a medium bowl.

3. Place parchment paper on a baking sheet.

4. Dip each piece of cauliflower into the batter and shake all excess batter off. Then place the pieces on the parchment paper. Repeat the process until all the cauliflower pieces are coated.

5. Spray the tops of the cauliflower with coconut oil cooking spray. Do this lightly by holding the bottle about a foot from the cauliflower.

6. Bake for 17 minutes.

7. While the cauliflower is cooking, melt the coconut oil in a small saucepan over medium heat. Add the hot sauce and stir. Once combined, remove the pan from the heat.

8. When the cauliflower is ready, put the florets in a heat-safe bowl and pour the hot sauce mixture over them. Toss to coat.

9. Place the cauliflower back on the parchment paper and bake for another 5 minutes.

10. Massage the kale until it is a bit wilted, about 5 minutes.

11. Place the kale in a bowl. Top with the Buffalo cauliflower and the Buttermilk Ranch Dip.

BELL PEPPER KALE SALAD

The only thing I ever really knew about kale growing up was that it was used at buffet restaurants as a garnish for more desirable dishes. With a little bit of education, I discovered that kale is actually one of the most nutritious greens you can eat. This nutritious salad has kale front and center, but it also has another healthy kick. Bell peppers contain para-coumaric acid, which is said to reduce your chances of stomach cancer. This salad is a win-win, for your health and taste buds.

MAKES 4 MEDIUM SALADS

3 cups chopped kale leaves
¼ cup Caesar Dressing (page 28)
½ cup raw sunflower seeds
2 tablespoons raw hemp seeds
1 cup diced bell pepper (red, yellow, or orange bell peppers work great, but use whatever you have)
½ cup green cherry tomatoes (or ripe cherry tomatoes)

1. Toss the kale and Caesar Dressing in a medium bowl.

2. Cover and refrigerate for 1 hour.

3. Plate and top with sunflower seeds, hemp seeds, bell pepper, and cherry tomatoes.

This salad is the perfect workweek lunch. You can make the salad the night before and take it with you for lunch, or chop the kale in the beginning of the week and make a salad every day by adding the dressing and toppings in the morning. By lunchtime, the kale will be the perfect texture, as the dressing will have broken down the kale.

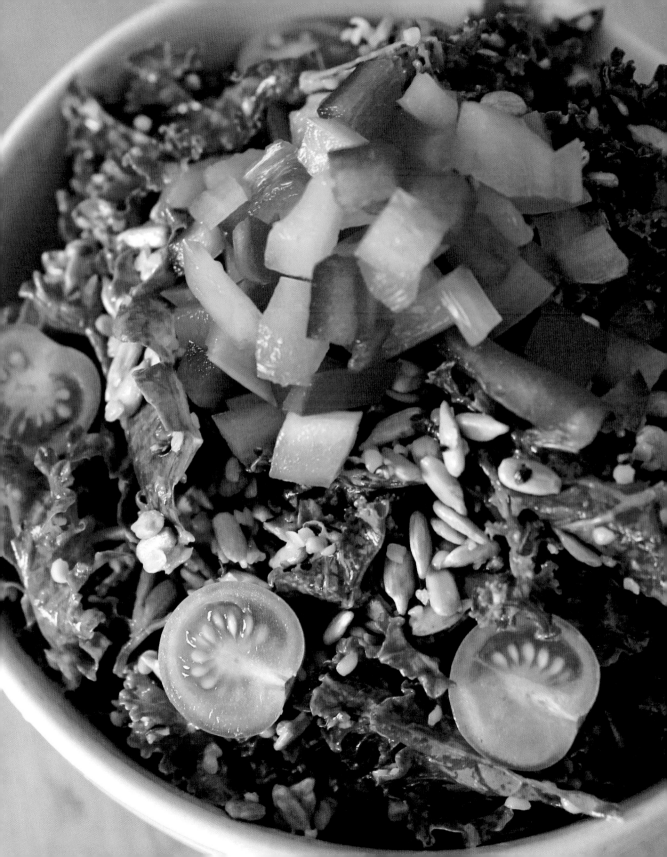

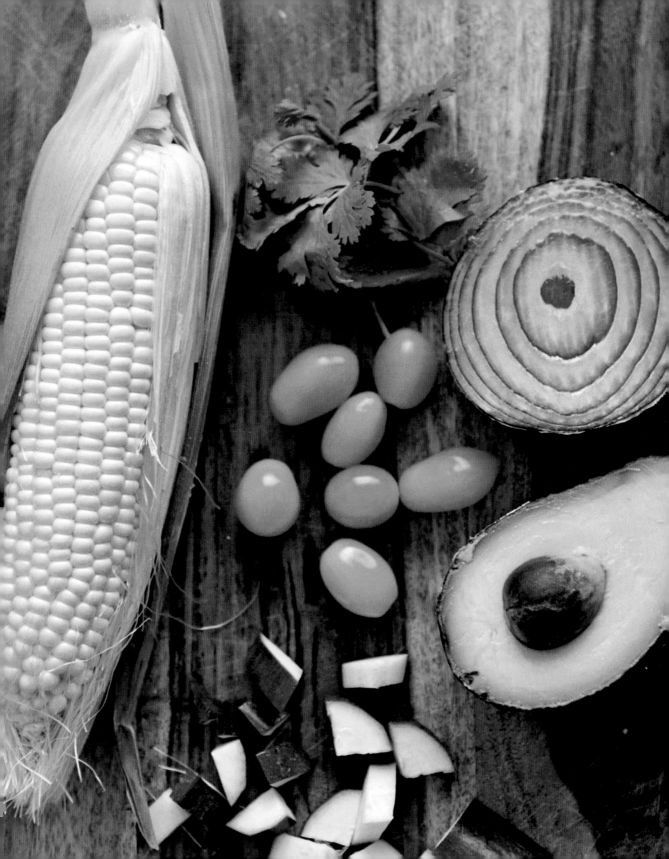

SUMMER SALAD

Salads can be salad without the leafy greens, especially when the farmers markets are overflowing with fresh corn, zucchinis, and tomatoes. This crispy fresh salad is my go-to side for barbecues, or a main dish for those hot summer nights when you can finally just open the windows and let a little breeze in by dinner.

MAKES 2 MEDIUM SALADS

1 cup cooked corn
3 zucchini, chopped
1 cup chopped cherry tomatoes
1 small red onion, thinly sliced
½ cup Cashew Cream (page 16)
1 bunch of fresh basil, thinly sliced
Salt and freshly ground black pepper to taste

1. Mix the corn, zucchini, cherry tomatoes, and onion in a medium bowl.

2. Toss with Cashew Cream Cheese or Cashew Cream.

3. Sprinkle with basil, salt, and pepper.

This is the easiest, freshest-tasting salad. You will never want to stop eating it! Feel free to add whatever vegetables you have lying around—carrots, beets, avocado—the sky is the limit!

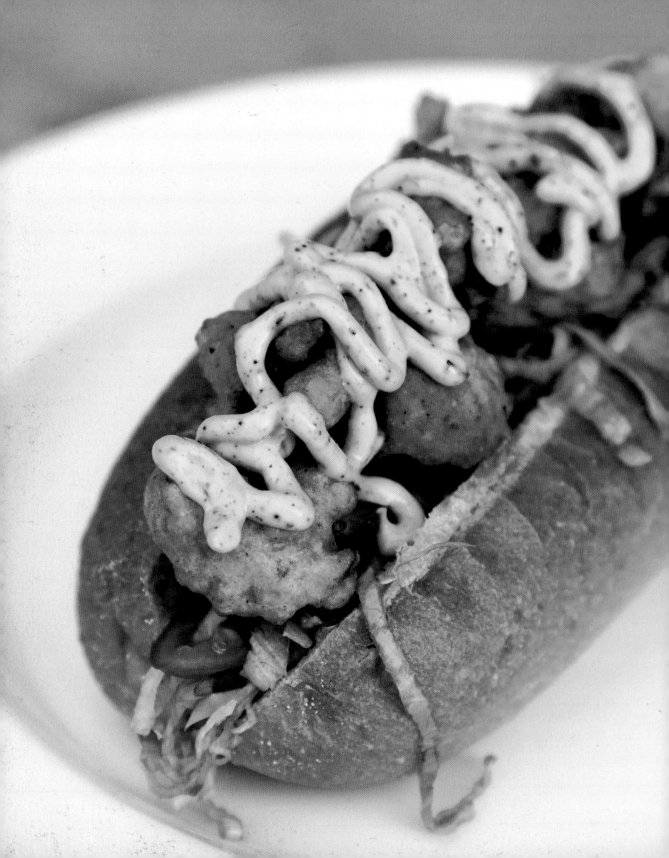

SANDWICHES

I promise you one day I will write a cookbook of just vegan sandwiches. I love sandwiches, and as soon as I went vegan they were the main thing I was excited to remake as plant-based. Who doesn't love a good sandwich? In this chapter, please trust me when I say you will not miss the traditional meat, poultry, or dairy in these sandwiches. Sure, the stereotype of a healthy vegan sandwich is a boring hummus wrap with some iceberg lettuce. But these recipes are far, far from that.

A quick note before we get started: *Always* use good bread. Ciabatta is my favorite, but if you can't find it at your local bakery, then Italian bread or hard rolls are great as well.

B.A.L.T. SANDWICH

(BACON, AVOCADO, LETTUCE, TOMATO, OR BETTER KNOWN AS THE BALTIMORE SANDWICH)

Named after the city that I love so much, Baltimore, the B.A.L.T. is a delicious vegan take on a traditional B.L.T. that doesn't mess around. The great thing about a sandwich like this is that you can eat it pretty much any time of the day. The combination of warm tempeh bacon mixed with the crunchy lettuce, sweet tomato, and creamy avocado is a magic no one can deny.

MAKES 4 SANDWICHES

1 (8-ounce) package flax tempeh
1 tablespoon pure maple syrup
1 tablespoon liquid smoke
1 teaspoon sesame oil
½ teaspoon smoked paprika
½ teaspoon ground cumin
½ teaspoon sea salt
4 buns, whatever type you like
½ cup romaine lettuce, chopped
6 slices heirloom tomatoes
1 avocado, pitted, peeled, and sliced
3 tablespoons vegan mayonnaise

 You can nix the vegan mayonnaise and the bun if you'd like! Avocado is creamy enough to take the mayo's place. Another variation: Instead of chopping the romaine, keep it intact and dice the tempeh—almost like a B.A.L.T. lettuce cup.

1. Cut the tempeh in half horizontally, then slice those halves into four squares.

2. Mix the maple syrup, liquid smoke, sesame oil, smoked paprika, cumin, and sea salt together in a small bowl.

3. Place the tempeh in a glass baking dish, then coat with the maple syrup mixture. Let the tempeh sit for 30 minutes.

4. Preheat the oven to 375 degrees F.

5. Cover the baking dish with aluminum foil and put it in the oven. Bake the tempeh for 15 minutes.

6. Remove the aluminum foil and bake for another 10 minutes, then remove the tempeh from the oven and let it cool.

7. Cut the buns in half and place the bottom halves on four separate plates.

8. Place the lettuce, tempeh, tomatoes, avocado, and vegan mayonnaise on each bottom bun. Set the top of the buns over the filling.

9. Cut down the middle and enjoy.

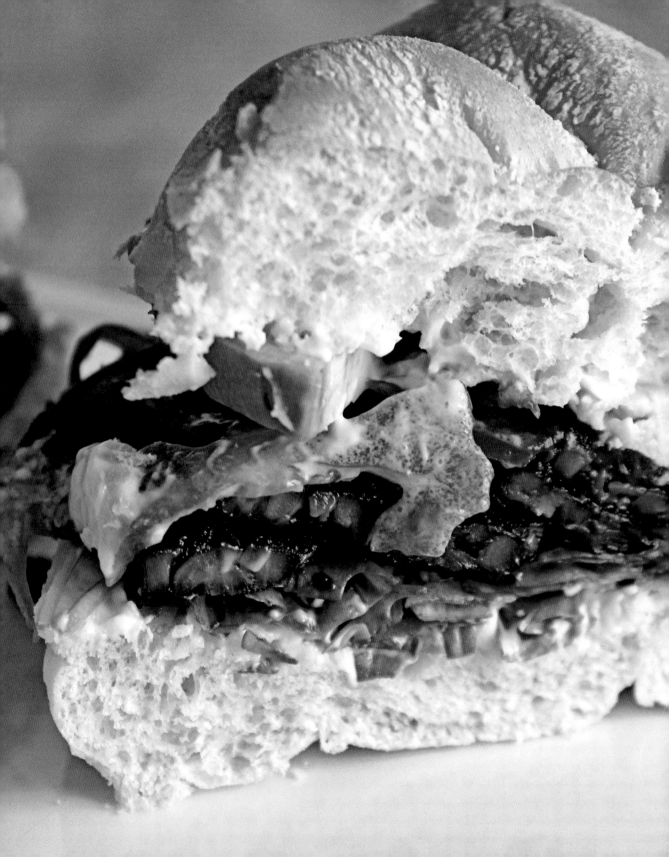

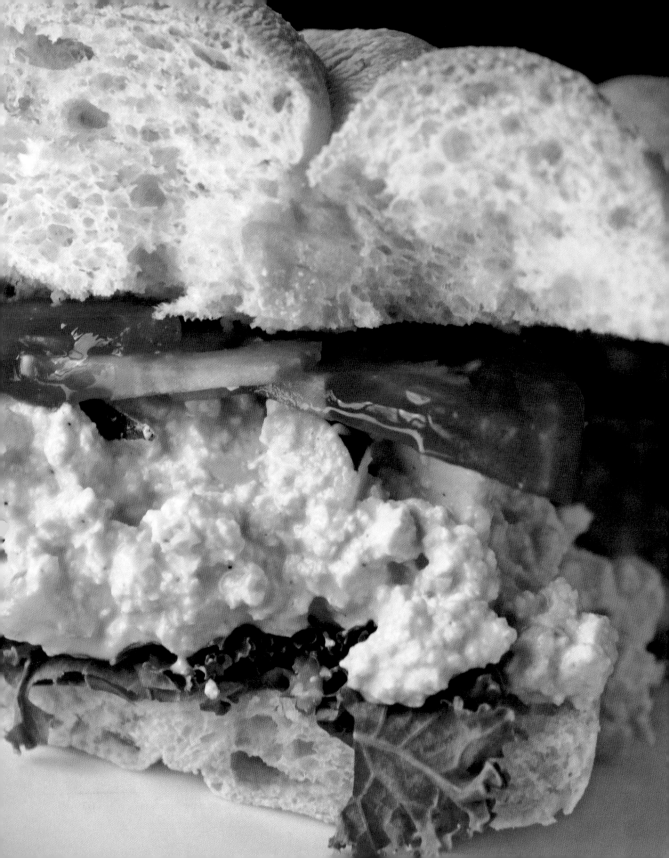

DEVILED EGGLESS SALAD SANDWICH

Using tofu as a substitute for eggs is something I've come to love over time. At first, I really only liked eating tofu fried. But then I realized that tofu could help me re-create something I was really missing: the taste and texture of a good egg salad sandwich. I was willing to try anything to satisfy that craving. So I put that extra-firm package of tofu to work and came up with a recipe my grandma would be proud of.

MAKES 4 SANDWICHES

1 (16-ounce) package extra-firm tofu, pressed
1½ tablespoons liquid aminos or soy sauce
1 tablespoon organic apple cider vinegar
1 tablespoon rice vinegar
1 tablespoon organic blue agave nectar
¼ cup diced celery
1 small red onion, diced
½ red bell pepper, diced
2 tablespoons chopped fresh flat-leaf parsley
¼ cup vegan mayonnaise
2 teaspoons garlic powder
1 teaspoon paprika
1 teaspoon ground turmeric
1 teaspoon ground cumin
1 tablespoon pickle juice
½ teaspoon kosher salt
½ teaspoon freshly ground black pepper
1 cup arugula or romaine lettuce
4 sandwich buns
1 tomato, thinly sliced

1. In a large bowl, gently toss the tofu, liquid aminos, apple cider vinegar, rice vinegar, agave, celery, onion, bell pepper, parsley, vegan mayonnaise, garlic powder, paprika, turmeric, cumin, pickle juice, kosher salt, and black pepper.

2. Cover with foil and refrigerate for 1 hour.

3. Place the arugula on a sandwich bun, then the eggless salad, then top with tomatoes.

You can also use romaine lettuce or cabbage leaves in place of the bread to make these gluten-free.

THE BEETS QUINOA BURGER

Quinoa is a great protein source. And what better way to get protein than in burger form? The texture of the quinoa in this burger complements the sweet beets well. Most people don't realize how versatile beets can be, but this recipe is a great example. These burgers can even get surprisingly crispy outside if you cook them just right. Patti Mayonnaise would approve. If you grew up in the '90s, you'll understand.

MAKES 5 BURGERS

2 tablespoons flaxseed meal
3 tablespoons water
2 cups quinoa, rinsed and cooked
1 cup peeled and grated raw beets
1 cup canned black beans, drained and rinsed
1 teaspoon smoked paprika
1 teaspoon ground cumin
¼ teaspoon ground coriander
½ teaspoon ground mustard seeds
1 tablespoon coconut oil
1 yellow onion, diced
3 cloves garlic, minced
2 tablespoons sifted unbleached all-purpose flour
1 tablespoon avocado oil

1. In a small bowl, mix the flaxseed meal and water. Let the flaxseed meal soak up the water for about 5 minutes.

2. In the bowl of a blender or food processor, place the quinoa, beets, black beans, flaxseed meal mixture, paprika, cumin, coriander, and ground mustard seeds. Blend until combined but not smooth.

3. In a large skillet, heat the coconut oil over medium-high heat. Add the onion and garlic and sauté them for 5 to 6 minutes, until the onion is translucent.

4. Place the quinoa mixture in a large bowl. Add the onion, garlic, and flour.

5. Combine the mixture with your hands. Form it into patties and place the patties on parchment paper. In the same skillet that you sautéed the onion and garlic, heat the avocado oil over medium heat.

6. Add the patties and let them cook for about 4 minutes per side, or until brown.

7. Place the patties on lettuce or on buns and serve them with arugula, sprouts, grated carrots, heirloom tomatoes, or whatever you have in your fridge!

 Don't forget to rinse your quinoa before cooking! Rinse it under cold water while rubbing the seeds. This removes the saponin coating that can cause quinoa to have a very bitter taste.

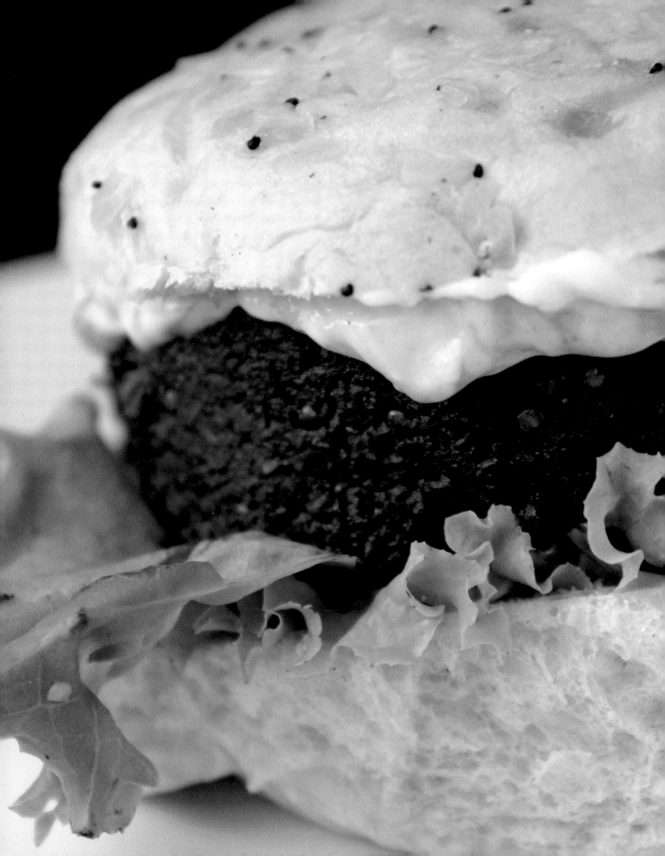

SHIITAKE MUSHROOM PO'BOY WITH REMOULADE

Po'boy sandwiches, the name of which is said to have originated from the term "poor boy," were made to feed workers on strike in New Orleans. Po'boys are one of the most satisfying sandwiches you will ever eat. They are traditionally made with fried seafood or roast beef. I decided to use shiitake for its soft texture. When I lived in Baltimore there was a creole joint down the street from my place that made the best po'boys I've ever eaten, hands down, especially the oyster po'boy. The shiitake mushrooms in this vegan version bring the texture of an oyster and the seafood seasoning brings the spice. Make this with my Black Bean Jambalaya (page 82) and beignets and you've got yourself some nice New Orleans cuisine!

MAKES 5 SANDWICHES

2 cups shiitake mushrooms, washed and patted dry

1 cup sifted unbleached all-purpose flour

1 tablespoon cornstarch

3 tablespoons baking powder

1 teaspoon garlic powder

1 teaspoon sea salt

1 teaspoon freshly ground black pepper

2 tablespoons seafood seasoning

½ cup unsweetened almond milk

½ cup water

1 cup peanut oil, for frying

REMOULADE

1¼ cups vegan mayonnaise

4 medium scallions, chopped

1 bunch of fresh flat-leaf parsley

¼ cup yellow mustard

1 tablespoon paprika

1 teaspoon Cajun seasoning

1 teaspoon horseradish

1 teaspoon pickle juice

2 teaspoons hot sauce

1 clove garlic, minced

5 sub buns

1 cup shredded iceberg lettuce

1 cup cherry tomatoes, halved

1. Coarsely chop the shiitake mushrooms.

2. In a medium bowl, mix together the flour, cornstarch, baking powder, garlic powder, sea salt, pepper, seafood seasoning, almond milk, and water.

3. Heat the peanut oil over medium heat in a medium, deep, heavy saucepan to 350 degrees F. Use a candy/deep-fry thermometer.

4. Dip the mushroom pieces in the batter and then place them carefully in hot oil.

5. Fry the mushrooms until the coating is golden brown, 3 to 4 minutes.

6. Remove the mushrooms with a slotted spoon and place them on a plate lined with a paper towel.

7. When all the mushrooms have been tried, turn off the heat for the oil.

8. To make the remoulade: Combine the vegan mayonnaise, scallions, parsley, mustard, paprika, Cajun seasoning, horseradish, pickle juice, hot sauce, and garlic in a blender and blend until smooth.

9. Place the mushrooms on a bun with lettuce and tomatoes. Top with remoulade and serve!

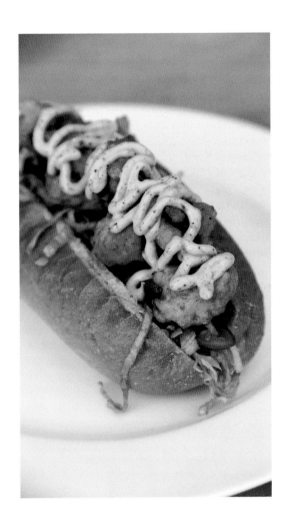

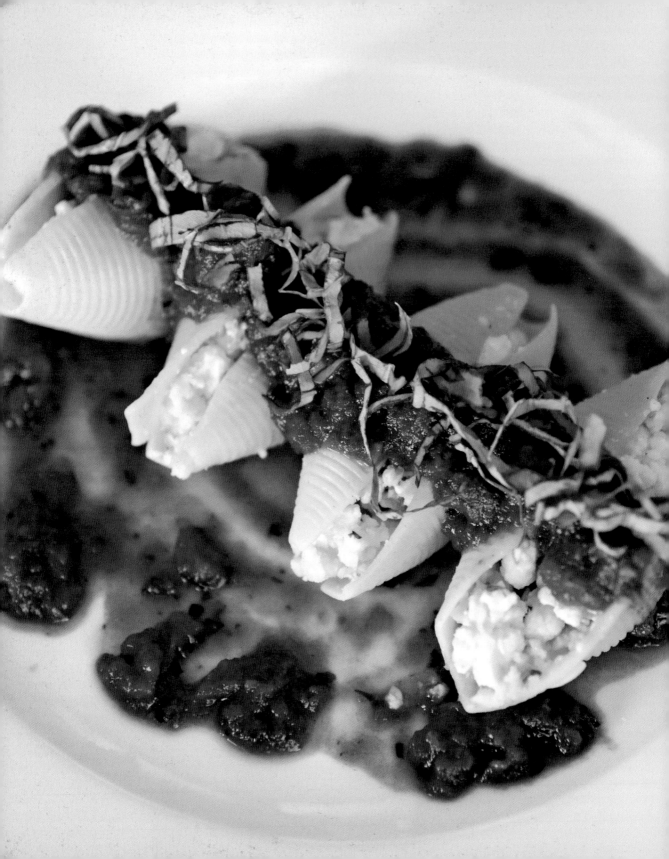

PASTA

Did you grow up eating spaghetti and meatballs for dinner almost every night, or was that just me? Regardless of your childhood relationship with pasta, it's hard to deny the comfort that a steaming-hot, hearty bowl of noodles brings. Loading up your pasta with veggies and the perfect sauce is key to a healthy, delicious, filling meal. Pasta is also the perfect blank canvas to help you explore new spices, vegetables, grains, and textures. And don't think you need to give up that creamy sauce you love—in this chapter you will find creamy sauces that will satisfy even the most cheese-and-cream-craving palate.

The combinations of pasta dishes are endless. And remember, recipes are made to be broken! Use what you have available in your kitchen or at the market. No zucchini, but you've got an eggplant on its last legs? Substitute away!

WONDERLAND ALFREDO

Just because you give up dairy does not mean that you have to give up the wonderful foods that you love. Wonderland Alfredo is a perfect example of that. Pour some wine or a nice glass of sparkling water and relax while you make this recipe. Sauce is supposed to be made with much patience and a whole lot of love.

MAKES 4 SERVINGS OR ABOUT 1½ CUPS OF ALFREDO SAUCE

1 box choice of pasta, cooked and drained, reserving
   ¼ cup pasta water
½ cup unsweetened almond milk
1 tablespoon rice flour
1 cup Cashew Cream (page 16)
1 teaspoon garlic powder
1 teaspoon dried parsley
½ teaspoon freshly ground black pepper
1 teaspoon salt

1. In a medium bowl, place the cooked pasta and pour the reserved pasta water over the pasta. Set the bowl aside.

2. In a small bowl, mix the almond milk and rice flour until the flour is dissolved.

3. Heat a medium skillet over medium-high heat.

4. Put almond milk–flour mixture in the skillet, then add the Cashew Cream.

5. Stir until the sauce is smooth.

6. Add the garlic powder, parsley, pepper, and salt.

7. Cook until the mixture comes to a boil, then let it sit for 5 minutes or until thick.

8. Place the pasta on a plate, then top with the sauce.

You can try this with gorgeous heirloom tomatoes or your favorite vegan sausage, too! This is the ultimate recipe to make for all your creamy-pasta-loving friends and family.

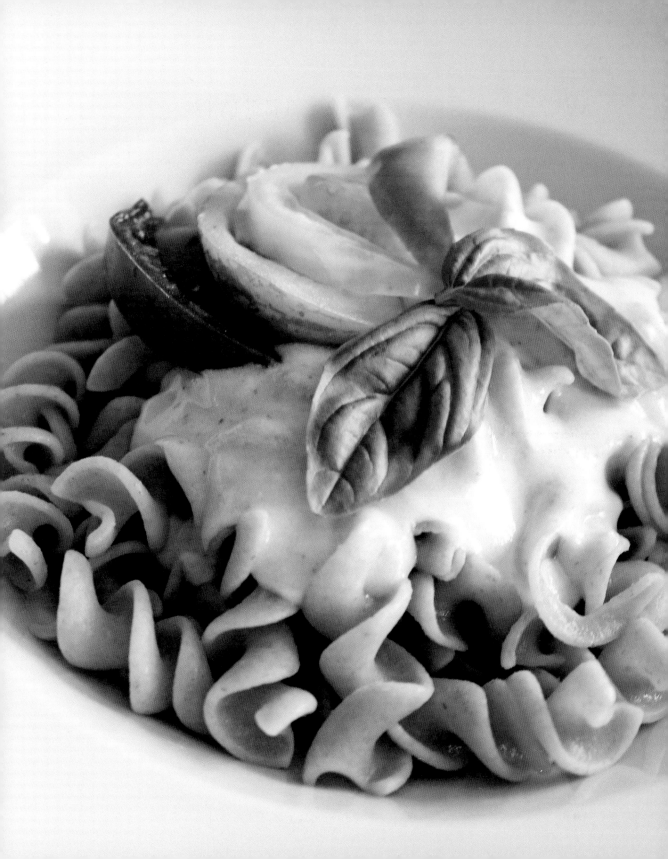

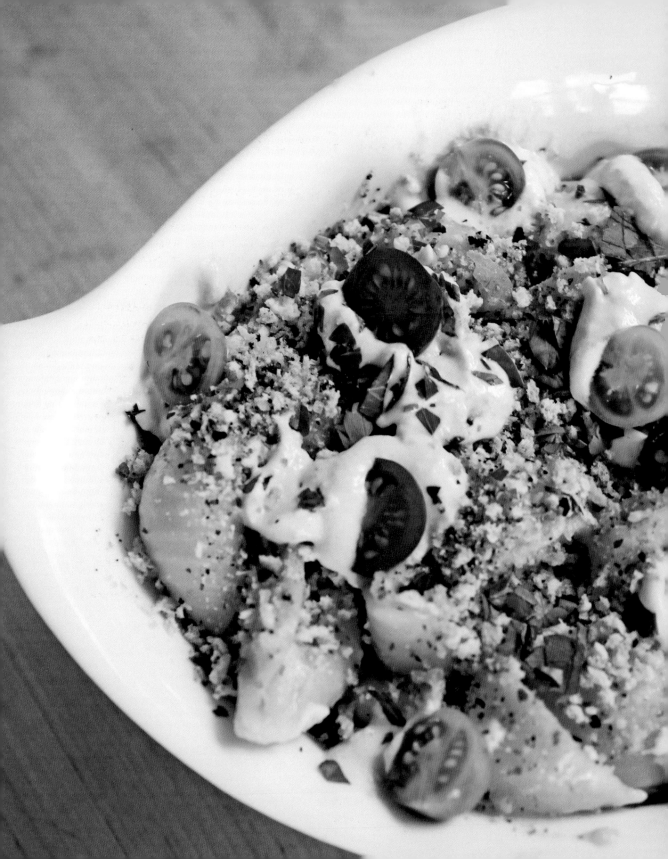

HALF-BAKED MACARONI AND CHEESE

The first thing people tell me when I say I am vegan is that they could never be because they love cheese so much. When I ask them what their favorite cheese dish is they say, "Macaroni and cheese," every time, without fail. So I made a dish for you to give those people, or make for yourself if you are one of those people. You don't need to give up your macaroni and cheese lifestyle for veganism. Embrace it, and enjoy this delicious plant-based version!

MAKES 4 LARGE BOWLS

1 tablespoon vegan margarine

2 cups unsweetened almond milk

¼ cup nutritional yeast

2 cups cashews, soaked and drained

1½ teaspoons onion powder

2 teaspoons garlic powder

1½ teaspoons sea salt

2 cups macaroni, cooked to al dente and drained

½ cup panko bread crumbs

1 bunch of fresh flat-leaf parsley, chopped

1 cup cherry tomatoes, halved

1. Preheat the oven to 350 degrees F.

2. In a blender, add the vegan margarine, almond milk, nutritional yeast, cashews, onion powder, garlic powder, and sea salt. Blend until the cashew cheese is smooth.

3. Place the macaroni in 9 x 13-inch baking dish. Add the cashew cheese and toss until the macaroni is fully coated. Save some cashew cheese to add on top while plating if you'd like.

4. Top with the bread crumbs and parsley.

5. Bake for 20 minutes. Remove from the oven and let cool on the counter for 5 minutes.

6. Top with cherry tomatoes and serve!

Use whatever macaroni you like best. Shells are my favorite because they're perfect pockets for cashew cheese. For a gluten-free version, simply substitute a gluten-free macaroni. I've found that quinoa macaroni works best for this recipe if you're GF.

MISS MARY MACARONI SALAD

This recipe is great for every BBQ. The first time I made this macaroni salad, I hid it in the refrigerator so that no one would eat it. I ate the whole thing within a two-day period. Breakfast, lunch, and dinner—I couldn't get enough of it. It reminds me of barbecues, pools, and Long Beach Island. Basically, it reminds me of everything that summer is. I can only hope that it reminds you, too!

MAKES ABOUT 5 CUPS OF MACARONI SALAD

½ cup vegan mayonnaise
1 tablespoon yellow mustard
1 tablespoon dill pickle juice
1 tablespoon organic granulated sugar
1 small onion, diced
1 teaspoon freshly ground black pepper
1 teaspoon kosher salt
2 medium carrots, diced
3 stalks celery, chopped
1 red bell pepper, chopped (optional)
2 cups gluten-free macaroni, cooked to al dente and
   drained

1. Mix the vegan mayonnaise, mustard, pickle juice, sugar, onion, black pepper, kosher salt, carrots, celery, and bell pepper (if using) in a 2-quart container with a lid.

2. Add the macaroni and toss to coat.

3. Cover and refrigerate for up to 6 hours. It will keep for up to 5 days.

N Don't forget to refrigerate before eating so the flavors have time to marinate and the sugar has time to dissolve.

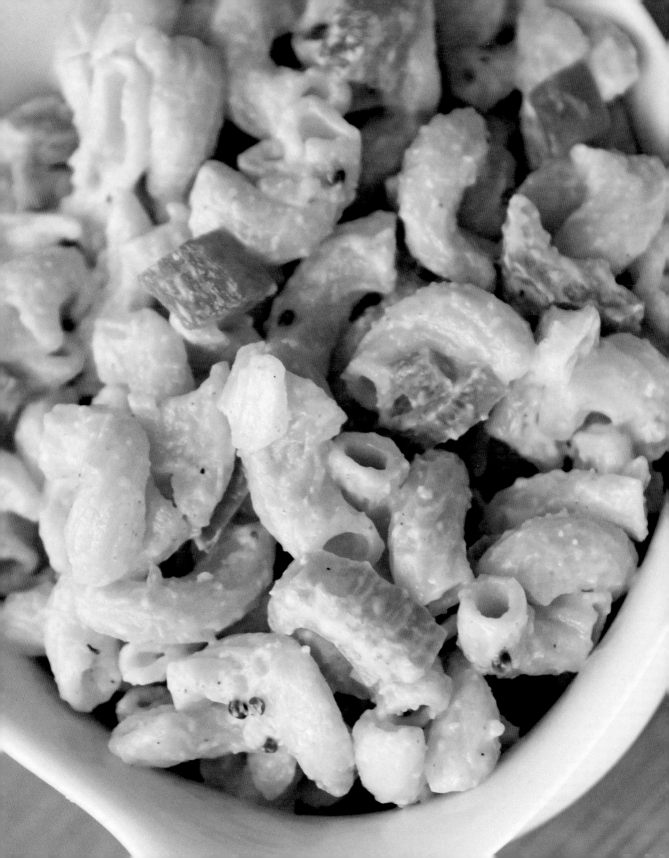

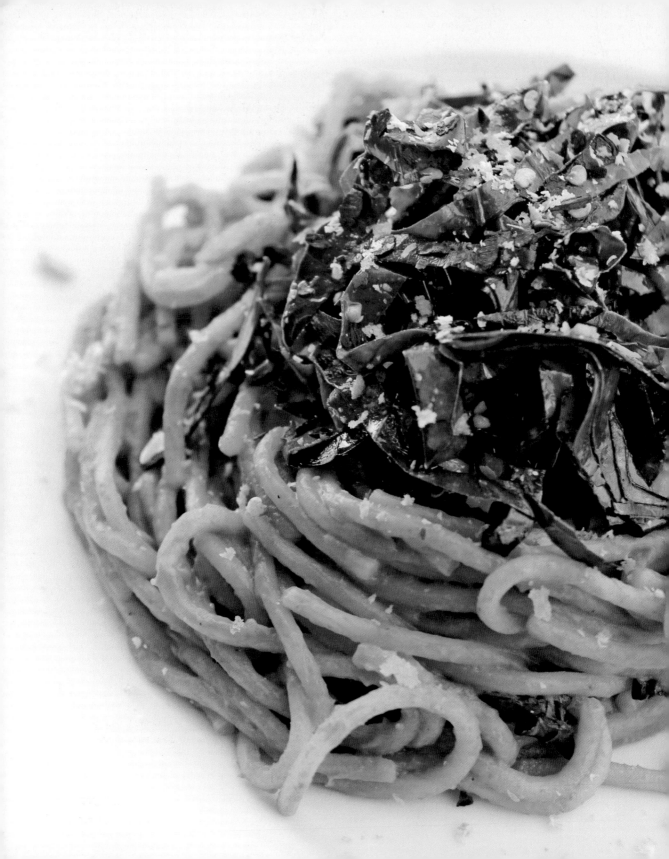

CREAMY BASIL TOMATO SPAGHETTI WITH KALE

You're probably thinking, *Kale? Again?* I swear, I'm not just trying to put kale where it shouldn't be. I love greens with my pasta. And kale is a great green to pair with a tomato-based sauce. Sometimes spinach gets a bit overrated. And adding new greens to your diet can be creative, with collard greens, Swiss chard, and kohlrabi.

MAKES 3 CUPS OF SAUCE

2 tablespoons coconut oil
4 shallots, sliced
4 cloves garlic, minced
1 (28-ounce) can chopped tomatoes
2 tablespoons tomato paste
1 tablespoon organic granulated sugar
½ teaspoon freshly ground black pepper
1 teaspoon kosher salt
1 cup raw cashews, soaked and drained
½ cup water
2 tablespoons extra-virgin olive oil
1 package spaghetti, cooked and drained
¼ cup coarsely chopped fresh basil
1 cup kale, lightly sautéed
1 teaspoon red pepper flakes
1 teaspoon nutritional yeast

 Strapped for time? No worries. Just buy a bottle of your favorite tomato sauce and use it in place of this homemade sauce.

1. Heat the coconut oil in a large saucepan over medium heat.

2. Add the shallots and cook until soft, about 3 minutes. Add the garlic and sauté for a minute.

3. Add the tomatoes, tomato paste, sugar, pepper, and kosher salt.

4. Simmer for 15 minutes, uncovered.

5. In a blender, add soaked cashews and water and blend until the cashews are smooth.

6. Add the cashew cream to the pot of tomato sauce.

7. In a large bowl, combine the cooked spaghetti and half the sauce. Toss until the pasta is well coated.

8. Add the basil. Then plate by using a ladle and large fork. Twirl a heaping amount of spaghetti around the fork. Place the spaghetti and the fork inside the ladle and continue to twirl. Once the spaghetti has formed a nice "nest," transfer the pasta to a plate.

9. Place the spaghetti on the plate and pull the fork up carefully (you may need two hands for this).

10. Pull the spaghetti from the center, making a nest-like shape. Add extra sauce to the center of each nest.

11. Place the sautéed kale on top of the extra sauce and sprinkle with the red pepper flakes and nutritional yeast.

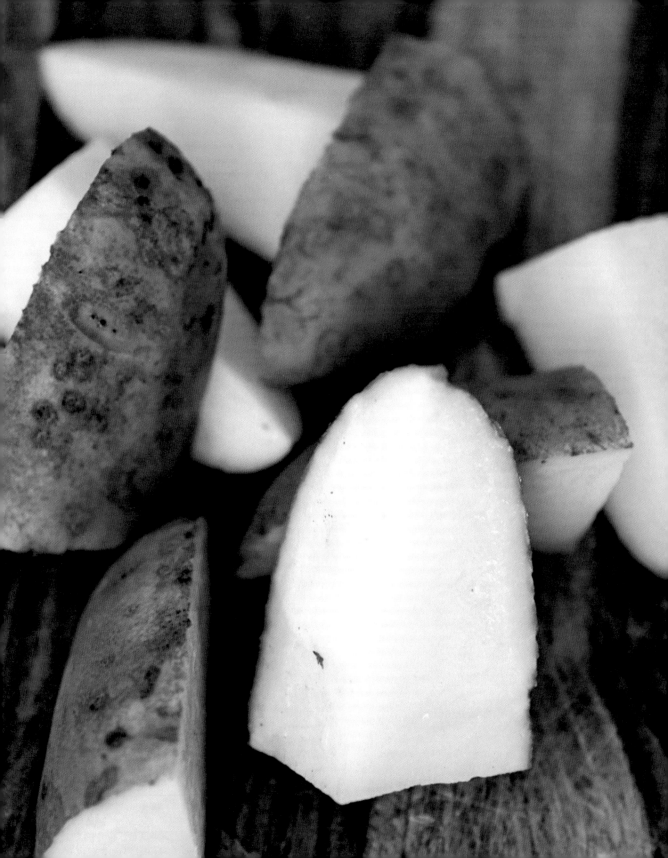

POKEY GNOCCHI

Have you ever been to a restaurant and gnocchi was on the menu, but you didn't want to order it because you had no idea how to pronounce it? Don't worry; I've been there. When I was teaching myself to cook, I learned so much about different dishes and their origins. It seems gnocchi was actually derived from the Italian word *noochio*, meaning "a knot in wood." Then again, some people say it derives from the word *nocca*, meaning "knuckle." Whichever it is, gnocchi certainly means delicious to me.

MAKES ABOUT 1½ CUPS OF GNOCCHI

2 pounds russet potatoes, peeled and chopped
1½ cups sifted unbleached all-purpose flour
1½ teaspoons sea salt
1½ tablespoons coconut oil

 Serve with Kale Pesto (page 22) or red pepper sauce.

1. Boil the potatoes in a large pot of salted water for 25 minutes.

2. Once the potatoes are tender, drain the water. Let the potatoes cool enough so you can handle them, then grate them into a large bowl.

3. Let the potatoes cool to room temperature.

4. Add the flour ½ cup at a time to the potatoes and mix.

5. Add the salt and mix together until the mixture forms a dough.

6. Place the dough on a lightly floured surface and knead the dough for about 2 minutes.

8. Shape the dough into a ball, then cut it into 6 equal parts.

9. Roll each piece into a rope about ¼ inch thick.

10. Cut the rope into 1-inch-thick pieces.

11. When all the dough is cut into pieces, press the tops of the gnocchi gently with the prongs of a fork.

12. Bring a large pot of salted water to a boil. Cook the gnocchi in the boiling water for 2 minutes, then drain the water.

13. Heat the coconut oil in a large frying pan over medium-high heat. Sear the gnocchi in the pan until they are light brown and the sides are crispy, about 5 minutes.

CAULIFLOWER RICOTTA STUFFED SHELLS

Cauliflower has to be one of the most versatile vegetables out there. You can fry it, blend it, bake it, sauté it, boil it (if you want your whole house to smell like cauliflower), and I'm sure there are some preparations I'm leaving out. Cauliflower also makes one hell of a ricotta-like filling for baked stuffed pasta shells. If you're not a huge stuffed-shells fan, just replace this pasta with some ziti and make some baked ziti instead. Remember, this is your kitchen. I'm just living on the shelf in it.

MAKES ABOUT 20 MEDIUM SHELLS

1 large head of cauliflower, chopped
2 tablespoons extra-virgin olive oil
¼ cup nutritional yeast
½ cup unsweetened almond milk
2 teaspoons garlic powder
1 teaspoon onion powder
1 bunch of fresh flat-leaf parsley, chopped
2 pinches of sea salt
1 (12-ounce) jar tomato sauce, or 1½ cups homemade tomato sauce
1 (12-ounce) package jumbo shells, cooked to al dente and drained

1. Preheat the oven to 400 degrees F.

2. In the bowl of a blender, blend the cauliflower, olive oil, nutritional yeast, almond milk, garlic powder, onion powder, parsley, and sea salt. Don't overblend. You want to eliminate big chunks of cauliflower, but you still want a coarse consistency.

3. Spread the tomato sauce on the bottom of an 8 x 8-inch glass baking dish.

4. Stuff the shells with the cauliflower mixture, arrange them in the baking dish, and pour the remaining sauce on top of the shells.

5. Bake for 15 minutes.

 Add some fresh basil and vegan Parmesan cheese on top if you have it! If you don't have shells, you can also use manicotti, or use the cauliflower ricotta for lasagna.

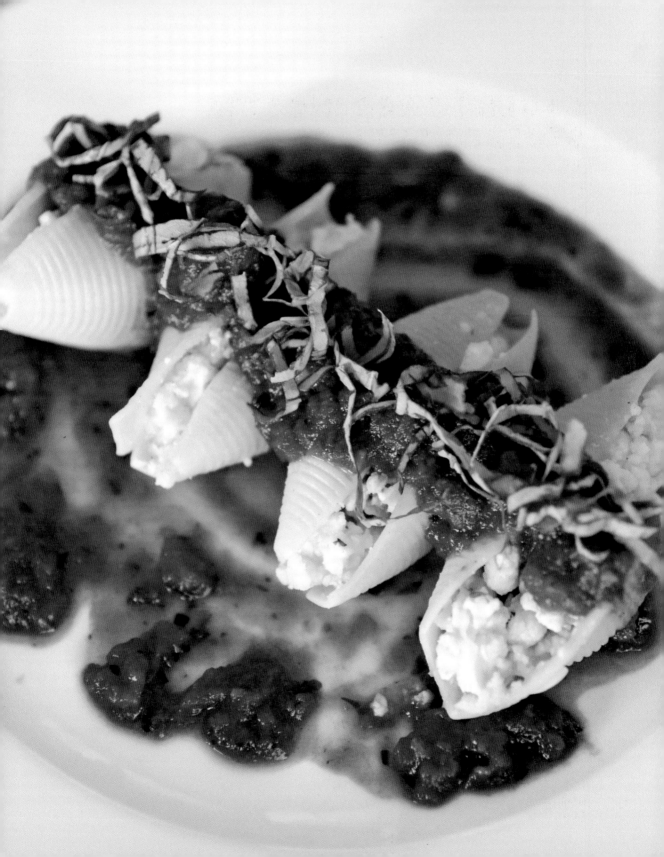

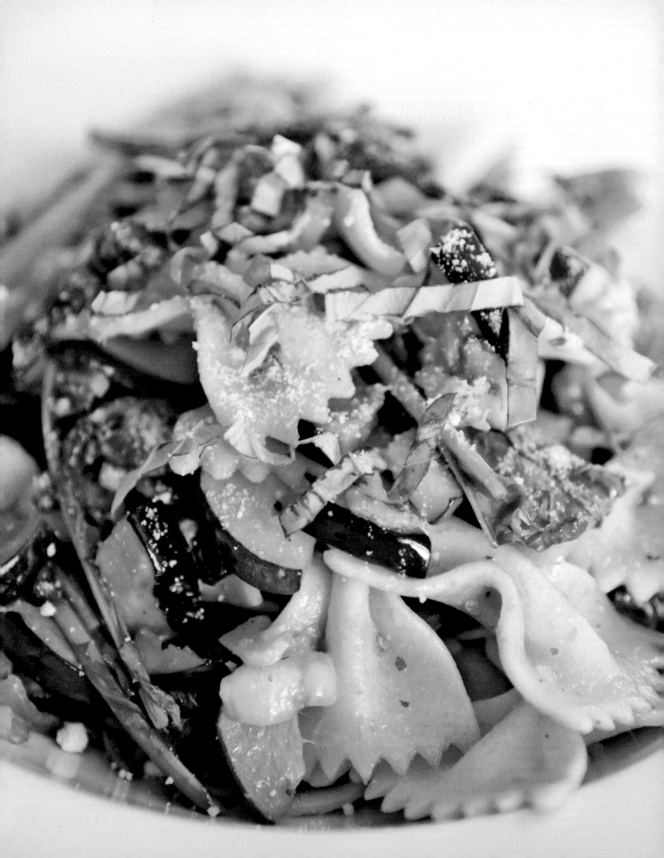

FIREFIGHTER'S BOW TIES

My brother-in-law, Matt, is a firefighter in New York City. What some people don't know is that most firefighters are really great cooks because they need to cook for their firehouse. Matt loves to be creative when he comes up with meals at the house, so one day, while we were at the market, we decided to veganize one of his favorite dishes to make with his coworkers. This bow tie pasta is usually made with meat, but we've created a hearty veggie version fit for hardworking, hungry firemen.

MAKES 4 LARGE PLATES

½ cup extra-virgin olive oil
4 cloves garlic, minced
5 medium sun-dried tomatoes, diced
1 small eggplant, chopped
2 zucchini, chopped
1 (14½-ounce) package bow tie pasta, cooked to
  al dente
1 cup chopped arugula
1 tablespoon chopped fresh rosemary
1 tablespoon chopped fresh oregano
⅓ cup chopped fresh flat-leaf parsley
1 teaspoon sea salt
½ teaspoon freshly ground black pepper
3 tablespoons finely chopped cashews
⅓ cup nutritional yeast
1 bunch of fresh basil, finely chopped

1. Heat the olive oil in a large skillet over low heat.

2. Add the garlic, sun-dried tomatoes, eggplant, and zucchini and sauté.

3. Remove the skillet from the heat and add the pasta and arugula.

4. Add the rosemary, oregano, parsley, sea salt, and pepper.

5. Plate, then sprinkle with the cashews, nutritional yeast, and basil.

N If you have some black olives lying around, you can throw them in, too, for a saltier pasta. I like to make this pasta on nights when I don't have time to make sauce and want something a little lighter.

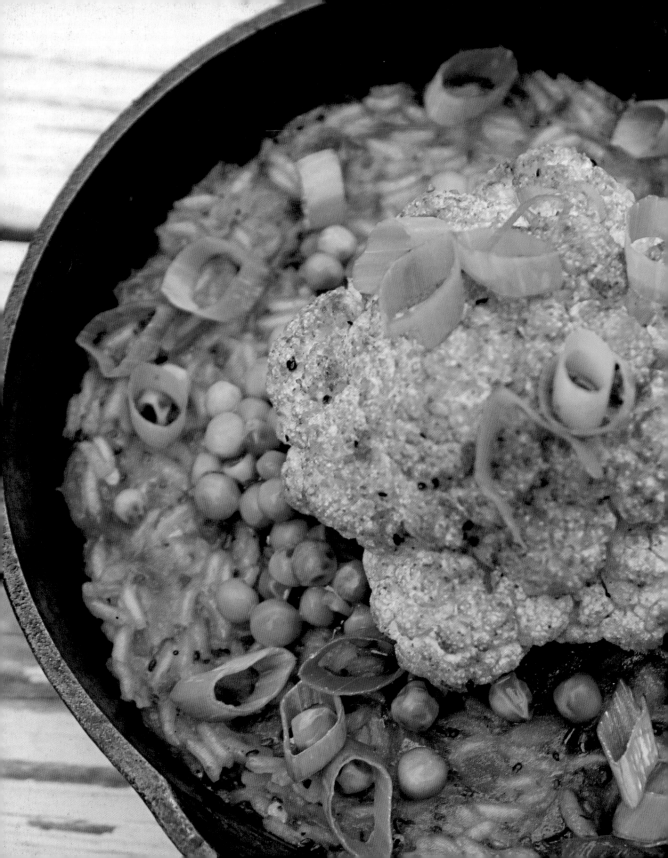

ENTRÉES

Sometimes when I tell people that I'm vegan, they look at me sympathetically and say, "So, you just eat vegetables for dinner every day?" Or, my favorite: "But where do you get your protein?" These people just don't get it. They think that because I'm vegan, I live a life of deprivation populated by steamed broccoli or kale and nothing else. But I love these moments because they give me the chance to educate these people that vegetables are so much more than just a side dish to be dutifully finished before dessert! You can do so much more with vegetables than you ever could with meat. In this section you'll discover delicious ways to roast, sear, grill, bake, fry, and sauté vegetables—methods that put the vegetables into the starring role on the plate, where they should be. And I dare any non-vegan to eat my rich, hearty Mushroom Cauliflower Harissa Paella or my Cauliflower Steak and say they're not filling.

And once and for all: We get our protein from vegetables! Enough to not only survive, but thrive!

BALSAMIC GARLIC PORTOBELLO CHOP

One day I had my dad, who I call "Pops," over for lunch. While I was preparing this hearty dish for him for lunch, he made a joke by asking when the real lunch was coming out. I said, "Don't knock it until you try it." He devoured his mushroom chop and decided to go vegan. He has been going strong for six months now, and by the time you read this, I'm confident he'll still be sticking with it. See, my dad didn't know that vegan food could be as rich and as satisfying as the meat-heavy diet he was used to. He had a heart attack five years ago, so I knew I had to convince him. This delicious dish is how I did it.

MAKES 4 MUSHROOM "CHOPS"

¼ cup balsamic vinegar
2 tablespoons coconut oil
2 teaspoons garlic, minced
1 teaspoon onion powder
1 teaspoon freshly ground black pepper
½ teaspoon sea salt
1 teaspoon pure maple syrup
1 shallot, thinly sliced
4 medium portobello mushroom caps

1. In a small bowl, mix together the balsamic vinegar, coconut oil, garlic, onion powder, pepper, sea salt, maple syrup, and shallot.

2. Remove the gills and stems of the portobello mushrooms, then rinse them and cut off any excess edges the cap may have so they do not burn.

3. Place the marinade in large plastic freezer bag with the portobello caps, then refrigerate for 20 minutes.

4. When the mushrooms are finished marinating, heat a large skillet over medium-high heat. Place the mushrooms in the skillet.

5. Cook for 3 to 4 minutes per side, until the mushrooms are browned and soft to the touch.

6. Place the mushroom caps on a plate and top with whatever veggies you've decided to pair your "chop" with.

7. Drizzle the remaining sauce on top of the portobello chops.

 While the mushrooms are marinating, roast or sauté whatever veggies you've got hanging around, and/or make some mashed potatoes or Garlic Cauliflower Mash (page 154) to serve with your chop.

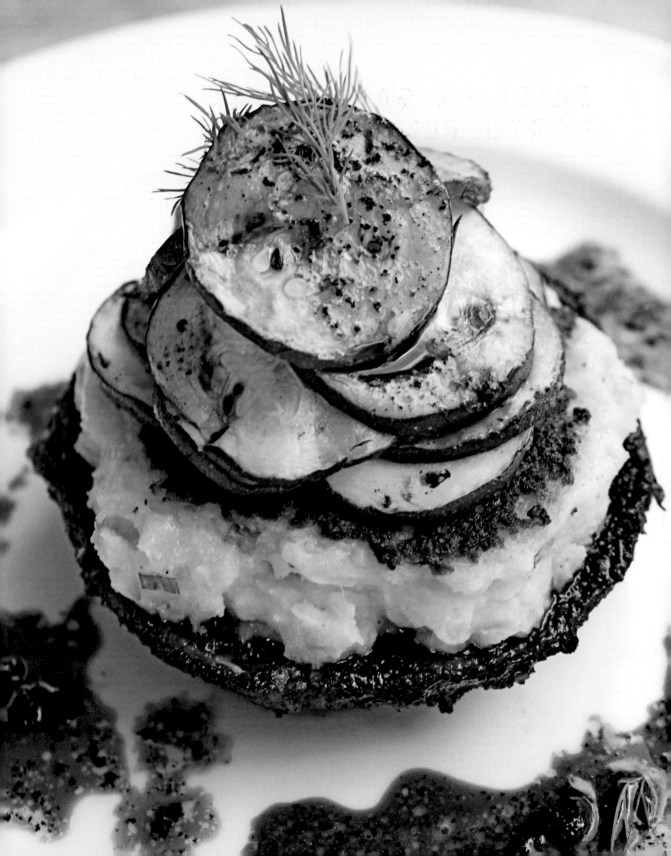

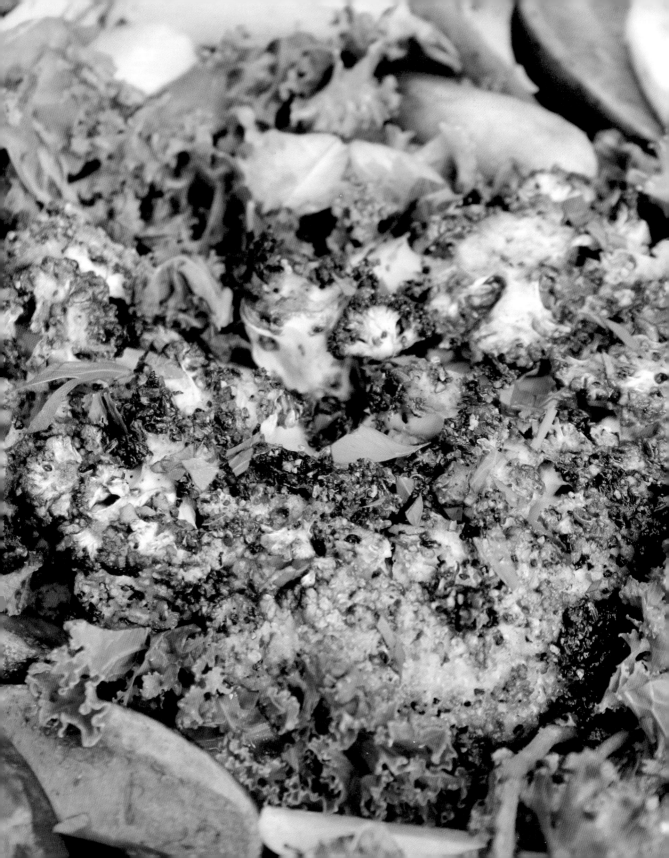

CAULIFLOWER STEAK

Cauliflower comes in many varieties, and I suggest you explore them when you make this recipe. The typical white-headed cauliflower you find in grocery stores is usually Northern European annuals. If you venture out to the farmers market, you are more likely to find different colors and varieties, such as white, orange, graffiti, purple, or Romanesco, that will make your dish more unique and colorful. Romanesco is the lime green cauliflower with pointed cauliflower curds. It's become more popular in the United States, and you should absolutely give it a try if you're lucky enough to come across it at the market. Don't be afraid to cook with a vegetable you've never cooked with before or try a technique you've never used. It's great to step outside of your comfort zone sometimes, especially in the kitchen!

MAKES 4 CAULIFLOWER STEAKS

1 large head of cauliflower
1 tablespoon freshly ground black pepper
1 teaspoon sea salt
1 tablespoon garlic powder
1 teaspoon chili powder
1 teaspoon ground coriander
2 tablespoons dry mustard powder
1 teaspoon dried oregano
1 teaspoon dried parsley
¼ cup coconut oil

1. Preheat the oven to 400 degrees F.

2. Cut the stem off the cauliflower and discard.

3. In a large bowl, mix together the pepper, salt, garlic powder, chili powder, coriander, dry mustard, oregano, parsley, and coconut oil.

4. Rub the cauliflower with the spice mix and place the cauliflower on a baking sheet lined with parchment paper.

5. Bake for 20 minutes or until the cauliflower has browned and formed a bit of a crust.

6. Cut the cauliflower into four slices and serve!

 Serve with roasted potatoes, radish, and kale. For extra-crispy cauliflower, bake it in a cast-iron skillet.

CRABBY HEART CAKES

I was never a huge fan of eating crab out of its shell, even before becoming vegan. I was, however, a fan of eating crab cakes. I didn't even know it was possible to make a vegan version, but then a friend of mine in Baltimore introduced me to hearts of palm. If anyone was going to figure out a vegan version of crab cakes, I knew I could count on a Baltimorean to show me his secret. Since then I've made multiple versions, and none are as satisfying and as decadent as this recipe.

MAKES ABOUT 10 MEDIUM CRAB CAKES

½ tablespoon coconut oil
½ cup minced yellow onion
½ medium red bell pepper, diced
2 stalks celery, diced
2 cloves garlic, minced
1 cup finely diced hearts of palm
2 tablespoons vegan mayonnaise
1½ tablespoons all-purpose flour
2 tablespoons seafood seasoning
1 teaspoon sea salt
½ teaspoon freshly ground black pepper
1 teaspoon chopped fresh flat-leaf parsley
1 cup sifted unbleached all-purpose flour
1 cup unsweetened almond milk
1 cup bread crumbs
½ cup vegetable oil, for frying

1. In a large skillet, heat the coconut oil over medium heat. Add the onion and sauté until soft, 4 to 5 minutes.

2. In a small bowl, mix the bell pepper, celery, garlic, hearts of palm, vegan mayonnaise, flour, seafood seasoning, sea salt, black pepper, and parsley.

3. Place the flour, almond milk, and bread crumbs in three separate bowls.

4. Take a palm full of the "crabby" mixture and form it into a patty.

5. Dip the cakes in the flour, then in the almond milk, then in the bread crumbs.

6. Place the patties on parchment paper.

7. In a deep skillet, heat the vegetable oil over medium-high heat.

8. Fry each crabby heart cake for 3 minutes on one side, or until golden brown. Flip the patties over and cook for another 3 minutes.

9. Place on a plate lined with paper towels to absorb excess oil.

 Serve with Tartar Sauce (page 29) and lemon slices on a bed of lettuce. If you're feeling fancy, serve up some succotash on top of the crab cakes instead.

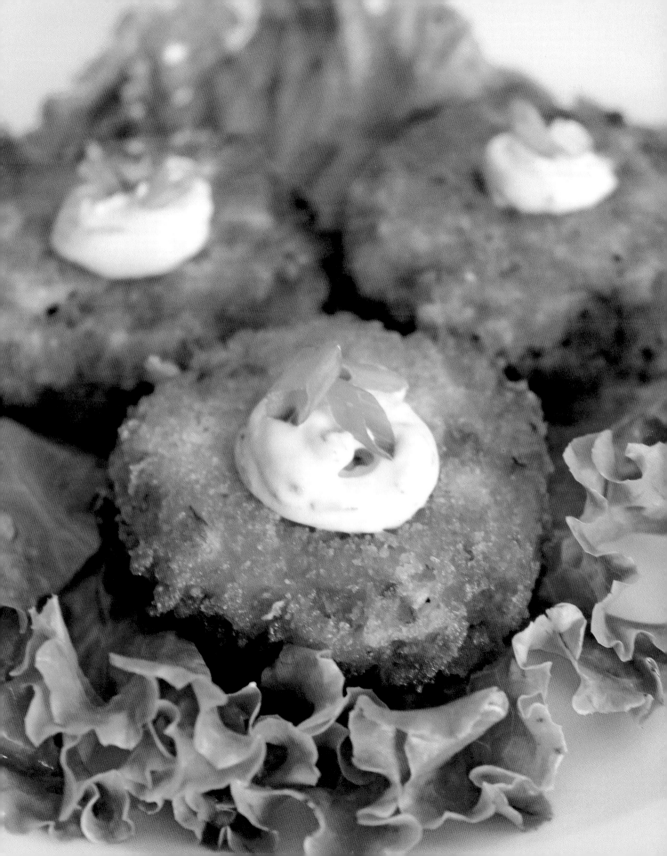

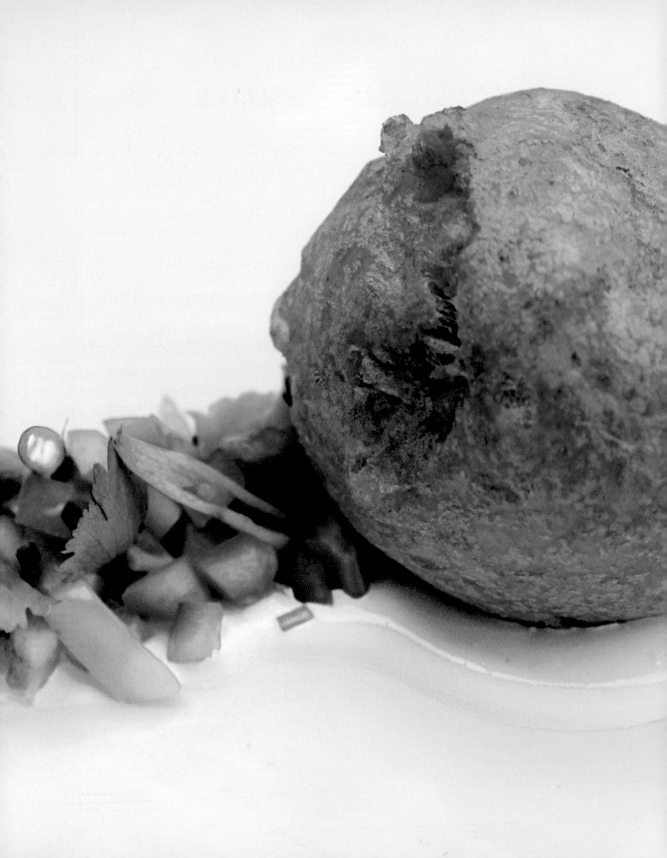

DEEP-FRIED GUACAMOLE

You've probably gathered by now that I'm a fan of frying things that you wouldn't normally fry. When I had some leftover guacamole one day, I decided that it was time for the avocados to get into that oil bath. The results were beautiful. Balls of food add a great dimension to a dish because they allow for room to neatly plate sauce or, in this case, sour cream. Just remember to handle them with care when you are forming and frying them. You don't want to end up with a bunch of guacamole with a nice heap of flour mixed into it.

MAKES 6 BALLS

4 ripe avocados
½ small red onion, diced
1 small heirloom tomato, diced
1 tablespoon garlic powder
3 tablespoons chopped fresh cilantro
½ tablespoon freshly squeezed lime juice
1 jalapeño, minced (optional)
2 cups sifted unbleached all-purpose flour
3 cups peanut oil, for frying
1 cup water
½ tablespoon sea salt

1. In a large bowl, mix the avocados, onion, tomato, garlic powder, cilantro, lime juice, and jalapeño, if using.

2. In a deep saucepan, heat the peanut oil to 375 degrees F. Use a candy/deep-fry thermometer.

3. In a small bowl, place 1 cup of the flour.

4. Take a handful of guacamole and form it into medium balls.

5. Gently toss the balls in the flour and shake off the excess flour so the balls are evenly coated.

6. Fry the guacamole balls in the hot oil for 30 seconds, then remove. Place on a plate lined with paper towels. Repeat the process until all the guacamole has been used. Don't worry, this isn't the finished product.

7. In a medium bowl, mix together the remaining 1 cup flour, the water, and the sea salt.

8. Dip the fried guacamole in the flour batter and fry in the hot oil again for about 1 minute, until golden brown.

9. Remove the guacamole balls from the oil and place on a plate lined with paper towels to drain excess oil.

 Serve with Coconut Sour Cream (page 18) and minced bell peppers. To make these hors d'oeuvres, simply make smaller balls and stick them with toothpicks.

KASHMIRI CAULIFLOWER AND LEEKS CURRY

Indian food always seems to have a laundry list of ingredients, which may seem intimidating at first. But you'll understand why they're necessary when you sit down to take that first bite. I tried to stay true to the traditional version of this Kashmiri dish as much as possible, while using ingredients you can find at your local supermarket. Have some family who haven't yet explored their curry dreams? This dish is for them.

MAKES 4 SERVINGS

1 medium head of cauliflower, leaves and stem
  removed
3 tablespoons coconut oil
2 large leeks, trimmed and thinly sliced
4 cloves garlic, diced
1 large yellow onion, diced
½ cup coconut water
1 tablespoon rice flour
1 teaspoon ground ginger
2 tomatoes, chopped
1 teaspoon freshly ground black pepper
1 tablespoon ground coriander
1 teaspoon ground cumin
1 teaspoon ground turmeric
⅛ teaspoon ground nutmeg
1 tablespoon red curry powder
1 teaspoon ground cinnamon
1 cup canned coconut cream
1 teaspoon sea salt
2 bay leaves
3 whole cloves
1 bunch of scallions, greens parts only, sliced

1. In a large pot, bring salted water to a boil over high heat and add the cauliflower. Cook for 7 to 8 minutes, until the cauliflower is tender. Set aside.

2. In a large skillet, heat the coconut oil over medium heat.

3. Add the leeks, garlic, and onion and sauté for 5 minutes, or until the onion is translucent.

4. In a small bowl, mix together the coconut water and rice flour.

5. Add the flour mixture to the skillet.

6. Add the ginger, tomatoes, pepper, coriander, cumin, turmeric, and nutmeg.

7. Cover and cook for 10 minutes or until the sauce begins to thicken.

8. Add the red curry powder, cinnamon, coconut cream, and sea salt.

9. Add the bay leaves and whole cloves to the top of the dish and cover. Cook for 10 minutes more.

10. Remove the bay leaves and add the cauliflower. Cook for another 5 minutes.

11. Top with scallions.

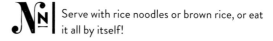 Serve with rice noodles or brown rice, or eat it all by itself!

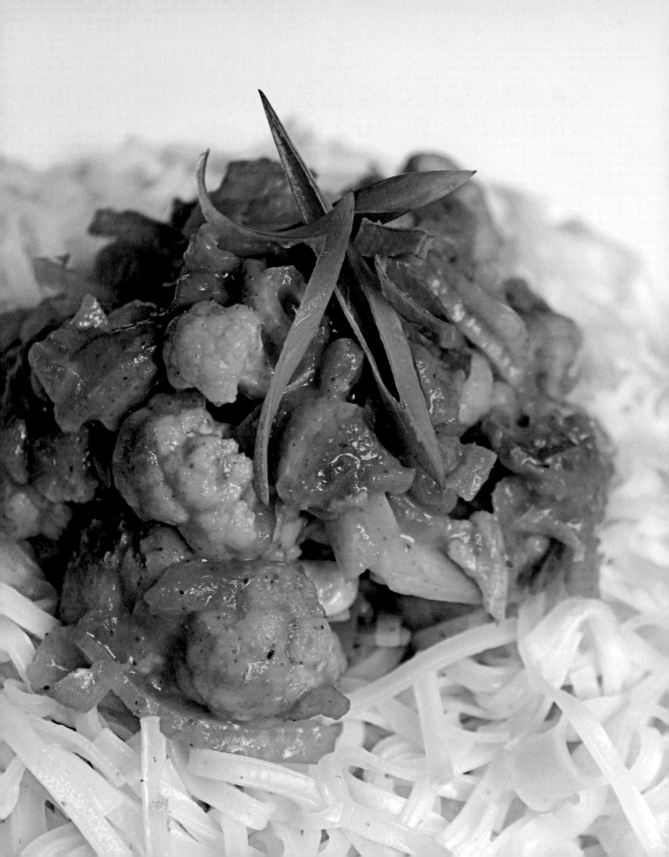

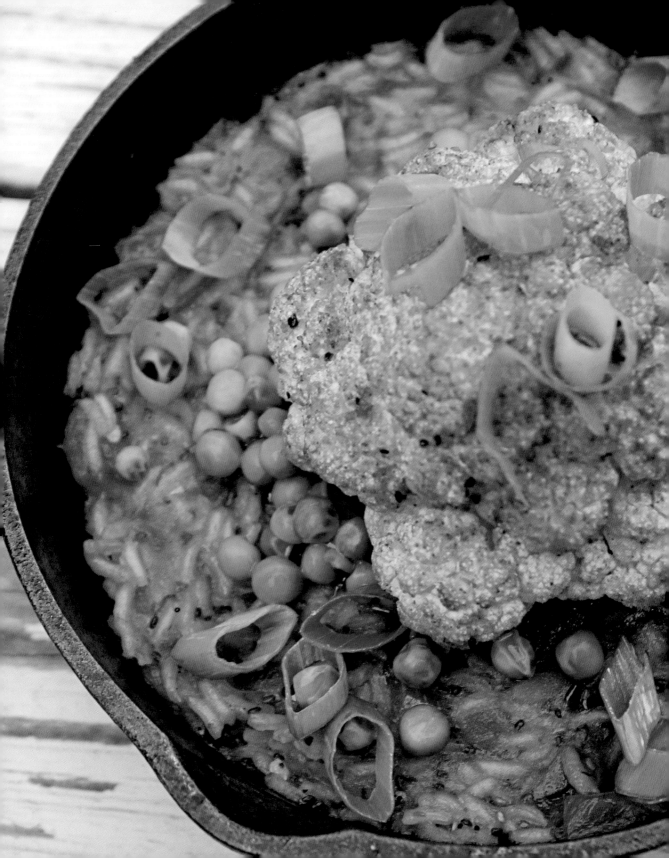

MUSHROOM CAULIFLOWER HARISSA PAELLA

Traditionally, paella is served with seafood and unlikely ever with harissa. But roasted cauliflower is a satisfying and very tasty alternative to seafood, and harissa adds a twist of flavor. You can't go wrong with many things that have saffron in them. Speaking of things you probably don't have in your kitchen, there's no need to stress over having a paella pan. If you aren't a paella maker and you'd like to just try it a couple of times, I suggest using a skillet. If you plan to keep making paella on the regular, a paella pan is a great investment for your kitchen.

MAKES 6 MEDIUM BOWLS OF PAELLA

2 tablespoons avocado oil
1 small yellow onion, minced
1 clove garlic, minced
3 cups Vegetable Broth (page 19)
½ cup canned diced tomatoes
1 teaspoon garlic powder
1 large pinch of saffron
1 tablespoon harissa paste
1 bay leaf
2 cups Arborio rice
1 small head of cauliflower, leaves and stem removed
2 tablespoons vegan margarine, at room temperature
½ tablespoon seafood seasoning
1 cup peas, cooked
¼ cup chopped scallion
1 lemon, cut into wedges

1. Preheat the oven to 400 degrees F.

2. In a large, deep, straight-sided skillet, heat the avocado oil over medium-high heat.

3. Add the onion and garlic. Sauté for about 5 minutes, until the onion is soft.

4. Add the vegetable broth, tomatoes, garlic powder, saffron, harissa, and bay leaf. Cook for 10 minutes.

5. Remove the bay leaf. Add the Arborio rice and mix until combined. Simmer for 20 minutes.

6. Meanwhile, place the cauliflower in an 8 x 8-inch baking pan.

7. In a small bowl, mix together the vegan margarine and seafood seasoning. Rub the mixture over the cauliflower until well coated.

8. Bake the cauliflower for 20 minutes.

9. Once the 20 minutes is up for the rice, raise the heat to high and cook for 3 to 4 minutes so that the bottom of the rice will crisp.

10. Remove the rice from the heat and top with cauliflower, peas, and scallions. Serve with lemon wedges.

SESAME TOFU TACOS

Mixing cuisines is possibly my favorite thing to do in the kitchen. When it comes to home cooking, there's no one there to tell you you're wrong. That was the case in my kitchen the day I made these tacos. I was craving tacos and Chinese food but couldn't decide which I wanted more. I settled on both. Although this recipe takes a bit of time, your patience will be completely worth it. The sweet sauce acts almost as the salsa would in a traditional taco. Use kale to catch any of the sauce that tries to escape.

MAKES 6 TACOS

¼ cup coconut oil
¼ cup cornstarch
1 (14-ounce) package extra-firm tofu, pressed and cubed
⅓ cup pure maple syrup
3 tablespoons soy sauce
1 tablespoon sesame oil
2 tablespoons rice wine vinegar
1 teaspoon ground fresh ginger
2 cloves garlic, minced
½ teaspoon red pepper flakes
6 corn or flour tortillas
1 cup chopped kale leaves, massaged
¼ cup shredded carrots
2 tablespoons sesame seeds
3 scallions, chopped

1. In a large skillet, heat the coconut oil over medium-high heat.

2. Place the cornstarch on a plate and roll the tofu cubes through the starch until they are well coated. Shake off any extra cornstarch.

3. Place the tofu in the skillet and cook for 7 to 8 minutes, until golden brown on every side.

4. In a small bowl, mix together the maple syrup, soy sauce, sesame oil, rice wine vinegar, ginger, garlic, and red pepper flakes.

5. Place the crispy tofu in a large bowl and pour the sesame sauce over it. Toss to coat.

6. Heat the tortillas over an open flame until soft, flipping with metal tongs.

7. Place the kale on the tortilla, then the tofu, shredded carrots, sesame seeds, and scallions.

 I like to eat my sesame tacos with chili mayo, which I make by combining 2 tablespoons vegan mayonnaise, 1 teaspoon chili sauce, and 1 teaspoon soy sauce.

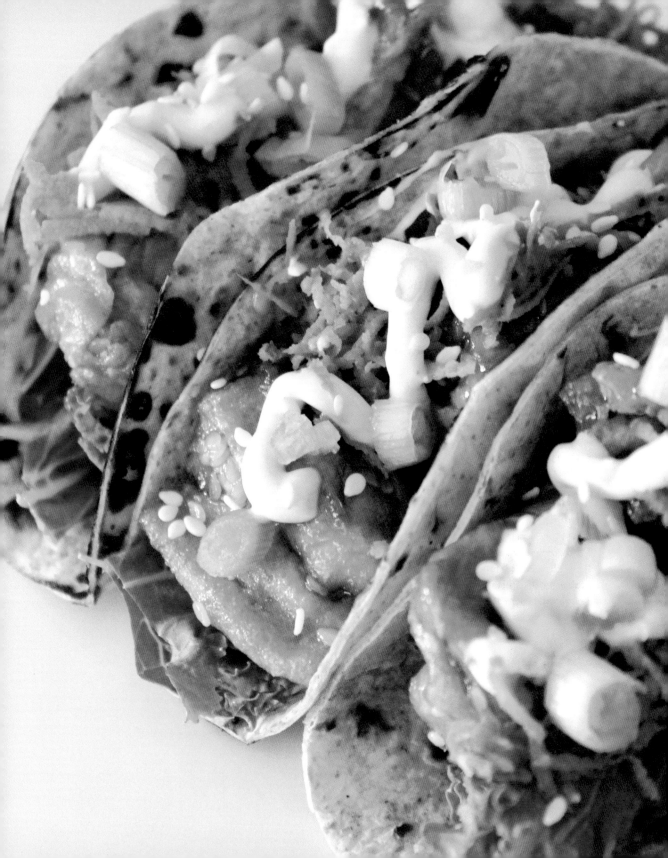

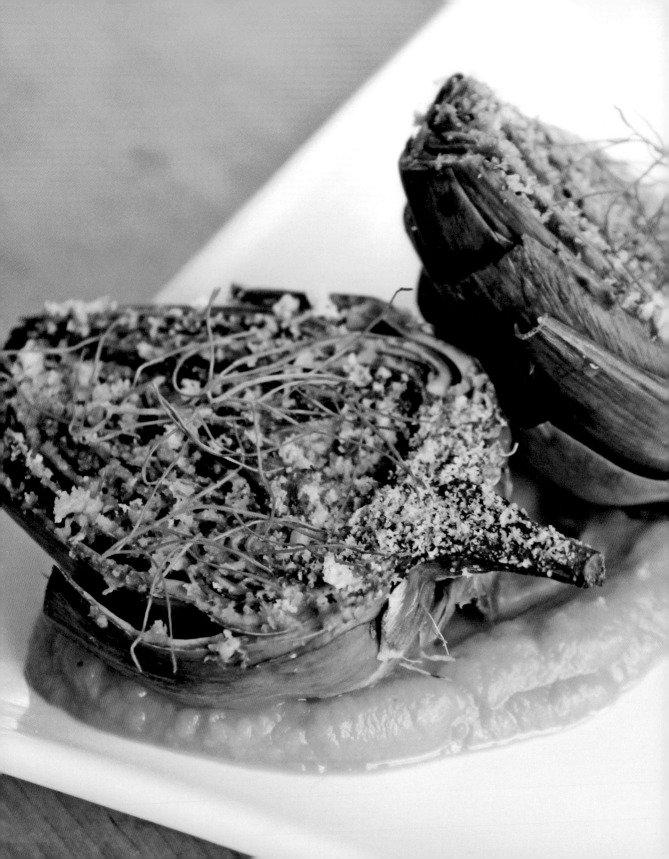

STUFFED ARTICHOKE

My nickname for the artichoke is "the Beautiful Disaster." You want to cook with it, but once you're halfway through trimming artichoke leaves, you start thinking, *How did I get myself into this?* If you've successfully roasted an artichoke before, though, it is probably your go-to "show-off" dish. The heart of the artichoke is enough to make anyone want to spend a little more time cooking these beautiful vegetables and a little less time complaining about them. My mom always tells me they're also more work to eat than they're worth, but I disagree. The act of pulling the leaves off and eating them and getting to the heart is an experience in itself. It reminds me of the tradition of eating crab with friends and family in Baltimore. It's an activity I no longer take part in, but it was always more about who you were eating with than what you were eating. This recipe allows me to get that tradition back.

MAKES 4 ARTICHOKES

4 large whole artichokes
1 lemon, halved
2 cups bread crumbs
¼ cup vegan margarine, melted
2 cloves garlic, minced
1 teaspoon onion powder
1 teaspoon chopped fresh oregano
½ teaspoon sea salt
¼ teaspoon freshly ground black pepper

1. Preheat the oven to 400 degrees F.

2. Trim the leaves of the artichokes with kitchen scissors so there are no more pointy tips.

3. Cut the stems down to about ½ inch.

4. Place the artichokes on their sides and cut them in half vertically.

5. Rub the lemon on the cut sections and place the artichokes in a bowl of ice water until needed so they do not brown.

6. Scrape out the chokes one at a time to remove and dispose of the hairs above the heart, then place them back in the ice water.

7. In a medium bowl, mix together the bread crumbs, vegan margarine, garlic, onion powder, oregano, sea salt, and pepper.

8. Pull the artichoke leaves apart and stuff with the bread crumb mixture.

9. Wrap the artichokes individually with aluminum foil and bake for 25 minutes.

10. Remove the foil and place the artichokes on a baking sheet.

11. Bake for another 10 minutes, or until the bread crumbs are golden brown.

MUSHROOM CHIA RISOTTO

If you've been vegan for some time now and have eaten at a restaurant that serves meat and dairy, you're probably accustomed to asking the waiter if the chef could make you something that you can eat. Nine out of ten times the waiter will come back and suggest, "Risotto." It has made me loathe risotto, but I don't want to. I loved it as a kid and I believe it should be just as good plant-based as it is with dairy butter in it. So I created this Mushroom Chia Risotto to give me the decadent risotto I've been craving. Chia seeds are an excellent source of protein, and I love to sneak them into dishes when I can. They also give this risotto a wonderful, thick texture—you can even stack it on a plate instead of putting it in a bowl, if you'd like.

MAKES 4 MEDIUM BOWLS OF RISOTTO

2 tablespoons chia seeds
½ cup water
2 tablespoons vegan margarine
2 cups bella mushrooms, washed and sliced
3 large shallots, minced
1 clove garlic, minced
2 cups Arborio rice
⅔ cup dry white wine
5½ cups Vegetable Broth (page 19)
½ cup Cashew Cream (page 16)
1 bunch of fresh flat-leaf parsley, finely chopped

1. In a small bowl, mix the chia seeds and water. Set aside.

2. In a large, straight-sided skillet, melt the vegan margarine over medium-high heat.

3. Add the mushrooms, shallots, and garlic. Sauté the mixture for 3 to 4 minutes, until the shallots are translucent.

4. Add the Arborio rice and stir to combine.

5. Add the white wine and bring to a boil until the wine reduces by half.

6. Add the vegetable broth one cup at a time. Once one cup of stock has been absorbed by the rice, add the next cup, stirring constantly.

7. Once all the water has been absorbed, add the Cashew Cream and chia seeds and toss.

8. Plate and sprinkle with the parsley.

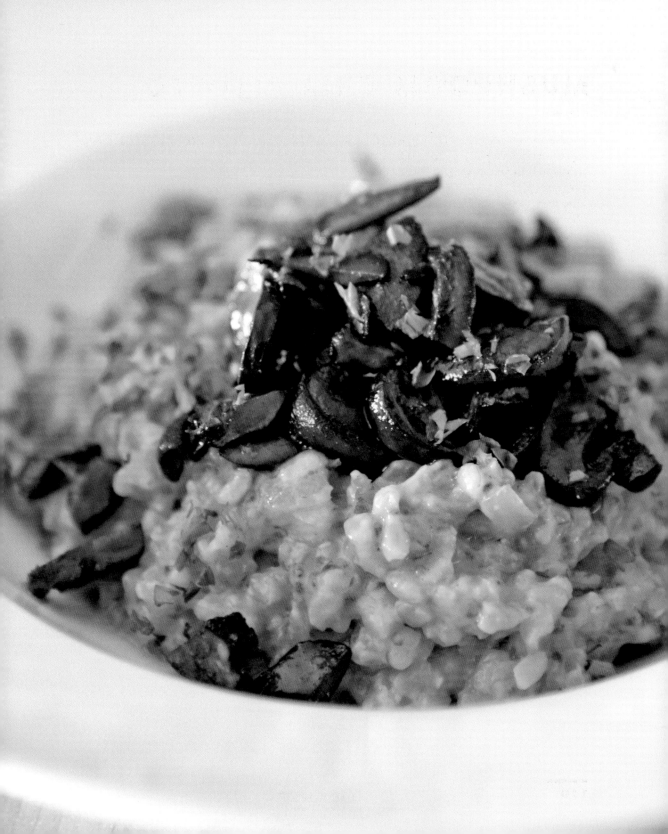

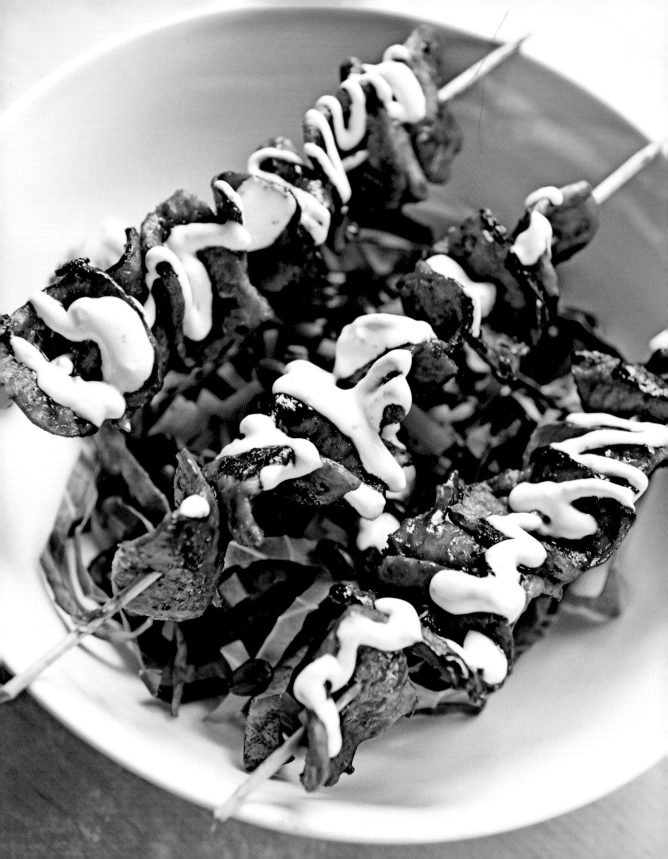

BBQ SEITAN SKEWERS

This recipe is not for the gluten-free lovers of the world, mainly because it consists of almost completely, well, wheat gluten. For those of you who do not have a sensitivity to wheat gluten but who are skeptical of the taste of seitan, I suggest you give this homemade version a try. Meat alternatives don't always have to be made by manufacturers who overprocess them. You'll feel a whole lot better about the proteins you're putting in your body if you're making them yourself. If this is your first time making seitan, or even hearing about it, don't stress. This recipe is super simple and easy. Vital wheat gluten can be found at most grocery stores and health food stores in the healthy foods aisle or baking aisle. Bob's Red Mill is my favorite brand to use. I recommend it for this recipe.

MAKES 8 SKEWERS

2 cups vital wheat gluten flour
½ cup nutritional yeast
1 teaspoon garlic powder
2 teaspoons onion powder
½ teaspoon ground cumin
5 cups Vegetable Broth (page 19)
2 tablespoons liquid aminos or soy sauce
1 small yellow onion, minced
1 clove garlic, minced
½ teaspoon kosher salt
½ teaspoon freshly ground black pepper
½ cup barbecue sauce

ALABAMA WHITE SAUCE
½ cup vegan mayonnaise
3 tablespoons organic apple cider vinegar
1 teaspoon cayenne pepper
1 tablespoon horseradish
2 teaspoons freshly squeezed lemon juice
Salt and freshly ground black pepper to taste

1. In a large bowl, mix the vital wheat gluten, nutritional yeast, garlic powder, onion powder, and cumin.

2. Add 1 cup of the vegetable broth and the liquid aminos and knead the dough for 3 minutes or until it is no longer sticky.

3. Form the dough into a long loaf.

4. Place the dough in the center of a large saucepan. Add the remaining 4 cups broth, the onion, garlic, kosher salt, and pepper. Make sure the dough is covered by the liquid.

5. Bring to a boil over high heat, then reduce the heat and simmer, uncovered, for 40 to 45 minutes, or until the dough is firm.

6. Preheat the oven to 400 degrees F.

7. Transfer the seitan to a 9 x 5-inch loaf pan and bake for 10 minutes.

8. Thinly slice the seitan and cut it into bite-size pieces.

9. In a medium bowl, combine the seitan and barbecue sauce and toss until well coated.

10. Heat a large skillet over medium-high heat.

(CONTINUED)

11. Stick the seitan on skewers, folding the seitan over to lessen the chance of it falling off.

12. Place the skewers in a skillet and slightly char each side, 4 to 5 minutes per side.

13. To make the Alabama white sauce: In a small bowl, mix the vegan mayonnaise, apple cider vinegar, cayenne, horseradish, lemon juice, and salt and black pepper to taste.

14. Top the skewers with the white sauce.

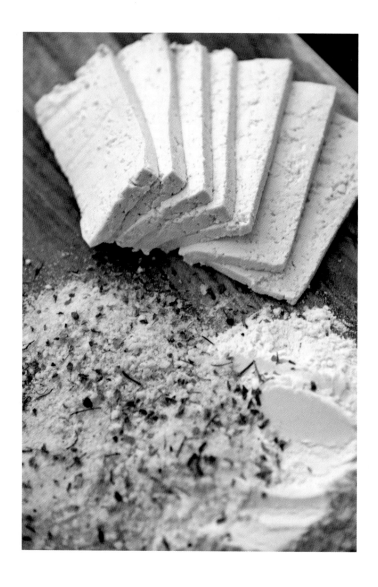

SOUTHERN FRIED BUTTERMILK TOFU

The perfect fried tofu always comes down to the batter and the texture of the tofu. The batter must be the perfect consistency, and the tofu must be firm and dry. They must be cooked in oil at the perfect temperature (360 degrees F) to get that crunchy outside that I love so much. Buttermilk is an essential part of an ideal batter, but not the buttermilk you're used to. How do you make a vegan buttermilk? It is as easy as 1-2-3. As you'll see in this recipe, it just takes almond milk, apple cider vinegar, and a little bit of mixing. Keep that in mind when making any recipe that calls for buttermilk.

MAKES 4 TOFU PATTIES

1 (12-ounce) package extra-firm tofu, pressed
1 cup sifted unbleached all-purpose flour
1 tablespoon cornmeal
2 teaspoons dried oregano
1 teaspoon garlic powder
1 teaspoon onion powder
½ teaspoon kosher salt
½ teaspoon freshly ground black pepper
1 cup unsweetened almond milk
1½ teaspoons organic apple cider vinegar
1 cup bread crumbs
2 tablespoons chopped fresh flat-leaf parsley
1 teaspoon chopped fresh oregano
Peanut oil, for frying

 Serve with sautéed okra, creamy collard greens, roasted carrots, and marinated beets. Top with your favorite BBQ sauce.

1. Slice the tofu into four pieces, then press gently between paper towels. Be sure not to press too hard. You just want to get the excess water out.

2. Set up three medium bowls next to each other. In one bowl, combine the flour, cornmeal, oregano, garlic powder, onion powder, kosher salt, and pepper.

3. In the second bowl, mix together the almond milk and apple cider vinegar until the milk curdles a bit.

4. In the third bowl, place the bread crumbs, parsley, and fresh oregano.

5. Once you have your bowls set, in a straight-sided skillet, heat about ½ inch of peanut oil to 360 degrees F over medium-high heat. Use a candy/deep-fry thermometer.

6. Dip the tofu into the flour mixture, then quickly into the buttermilk, and finally coat it with the bread crumbs.

7. Immediately place the battered and breaded tofu into the oil and fry until the bottoms are golden brown, about 4 minutes.

8. Flip and repeat on the opposite side of the tofu.

9. If the oil begins to smoke, reduce the heat.

CRISPY ORANGE SESAME CAULIFLOWER

If you've flipped through this book enough, you've probably figured out by now that I am indeed a sweet girl more than a spicy girl. So when it comes to Chinese food, I'd choose a sesame dish over General Tso's any day. This recipe is a vegan version of one of my favorite takeout dishes with a citrus twist. It is packed with so much rich flavor, you won't miss the world of MSG-sprinkled dishes (I say this only because I was addicted to the stuff). Plus, who needs takeout when it's this simple to make it yourself? Pairs perfectly with a romantic comedy on Netflix.

MAKES 4 LARGE PLATES

N | Serve over rice noodles, brown rice, or steamed vegetables. If you like to drench your plate in sauce, I suggest doubling the orange sesame sauce, especially if you'd like to eat it over the noodles, rice, or veggies you serve, too.

CAULIFLOWER
⅓ cup cornstarch
¼ cup sifted unbleached all-purpose flour
1 teaspoon kosher salt
⅔ cup water
1 teaspoon sunflower oil
1 cup vegetable oil, for frying
1 medium head of cauliflower, stemmed and cut into bite-size pieces

ORANGE SESAME SAUCE
2 tablespoons sesame oil
1½ teaspoons garlic powder
⅓ cup orange juice
½ tablespoon orange zest
2 tablespoons liquid aminos or soy sauce
1 tablespoon rice wine vinegar
2 teaspoons cornstarch
1 tablespoon (packed) organic brown sugar

CHILI MAYO SAUCE
1 tablespoon chili sauce
½ cup vegan mayonnaise

1 teaspoon sesame seeds
2 tablespoons thinly sliced scallion greens

1. To make the cauliflower: In medium bowl, mix the cornstarch, flour, kosher salt, water, and sunflower oil.

2. Heat the vegetable oil in a large skillet over medium-high heat. To test the oil, place a dab of the batter into the oil. If it sizzles without the oil splashing, you're ready to go.

3. Dip each piece of cauliflower in the batter, then place in the skillet. Do not crowd—you will have to turn them.

4. Keep turning the cauliflower until all the sides are lightly brown, then transfer to a plate lined with paper towels.

5. Once all the cauliflower has been fried, set aside.

6. To make the orange sesame sauce: Heat the sesame oil in a large skillet over medium heat.

7. Add the garlic powder, orange juice, orange zest, and liquid aminos and stir.

8. In a small bowl, mix together the rice wine vinegar and cornstarch until the cornstarch dissolves. Add the mixture to the skillet, then add the brown sugar and cook for another 3 to 4 minutes, or until thick.

9. In a large bowl, toss together the cauliflower and the orange sesame sauce.

10. To make the chili mayo sauce: In a small bowl, mix together the chili sauce and vegan mayonnaise.

11. Plate the cauliflower, topped with chili mayo sauce, sesame seeds, and scallions.

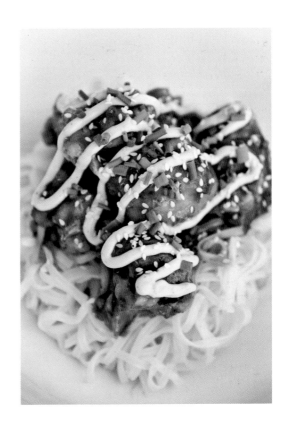

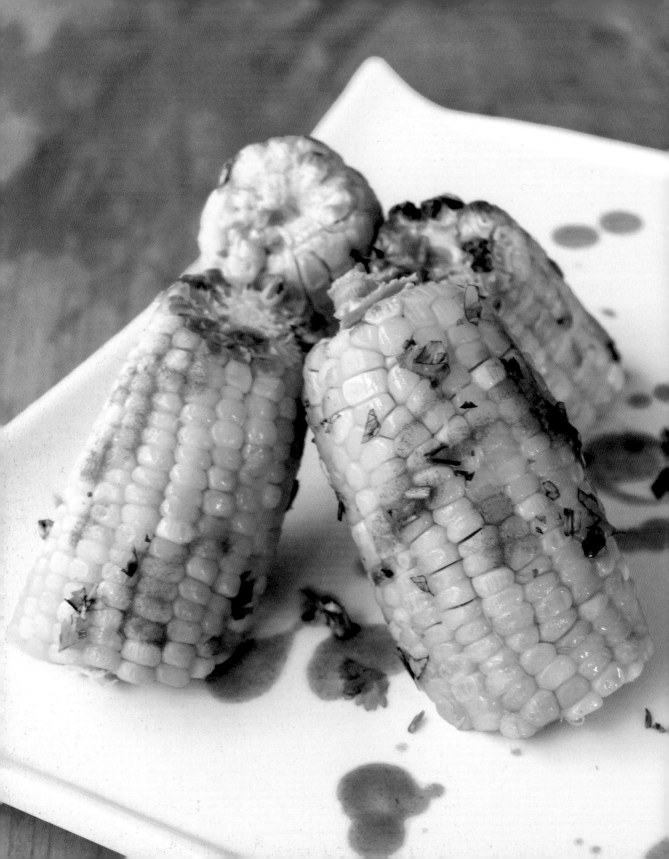

SIDES

The running joke in my group of friends when I first became vegan was, "Oh, Mary, what are you going to eat with your vegetables? Some more vegetables?" But they learned pretty quickly that I could eat pretty much everything that they could—and my sides were just as tasty, only healthier! Now my friends don't tease me about my extra veggies on the side—they want bites of my Buttermilk Biscuits and Pear Kale Slaw.

BUTTERMILK BISCUITS

Leave it to biscuits to remind you of a hot day down south. These soft, flaky, and delicious buttermilk biscuits are sure to fill all your Southern comfort food needs. Even though these soft round bundles of goodness are in the "sides" section of this book, feel free to eat them as a meal by making sandwiches out of them with some Southern Fried Buttermilk Tofu (page 145) and a drizzle of maple syrup in between.

MAKES 8 BIG BISCUITS

2 cups sifted unbleached all-purpose flour
½ teaspoon baking soda
1½ teaspoons baking powder
2 teaspoons organic granulated sugar
1 teaspoon sea salt
6 tablespoons vegan margarine
1 cup unsweetened almond milk
1 tablespoon organic apple cider vinegar

 Making dough can be a tricky task, but if you can master handling it as little as possible, then you're going to be a biscuit master. Just think of the possibilities: biscuits and gravy, strawberry shortcake, breakfast sandwiches—the list goes on!

1. Preheat the oven to 450 degrees F.

2. In a large bowl, mix the flour, baking soda, baking powder, sugar, and sea salt.

3. With a fork, cut in the vegan margarine until the flour mixture has become coarse.

4. In a small bowl, mix together the almond milk and apple cider vinegar until the milk curdles a bit. Then pour it into the flour mixture.

5. Gently flatten the dough with your hands until it is about ½ inch thick. Fold the dough over as many times as you can, then flatten again until the dough is about 1 inch thick.

6. Use a glass to cut the dough into rounds. Make sure you place the glass close to the last place you cut out so that you use as much dough as possible because the first-cut dough will come out better than when you knead the dough again.

7. Place the dough circles on a cookie sheet lined with parchment paper, about ½ inch apart.

8. Bake for 10 minutes, or until the biscuits are a light golden brown.

9. Keep an eye on these guys, as they will burn easily.

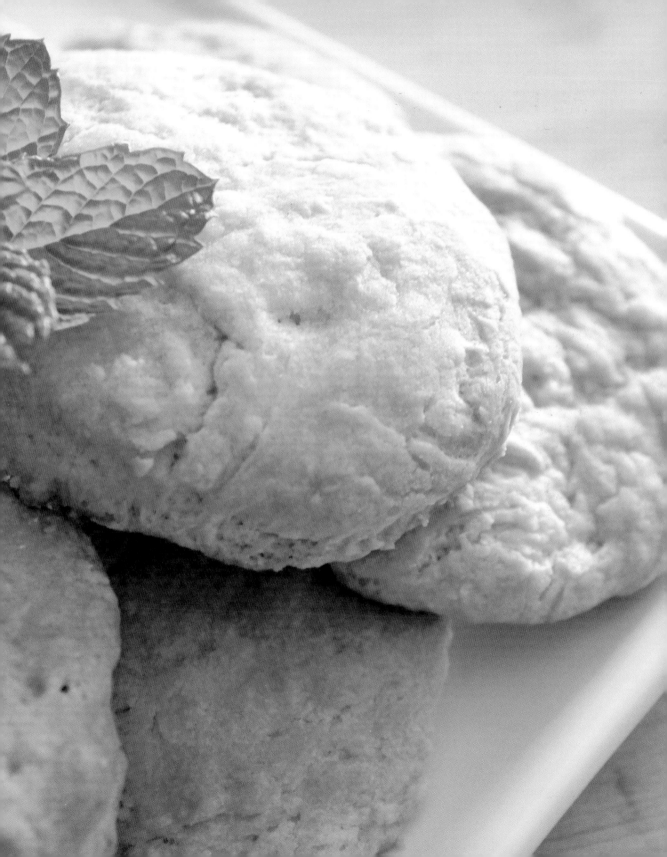

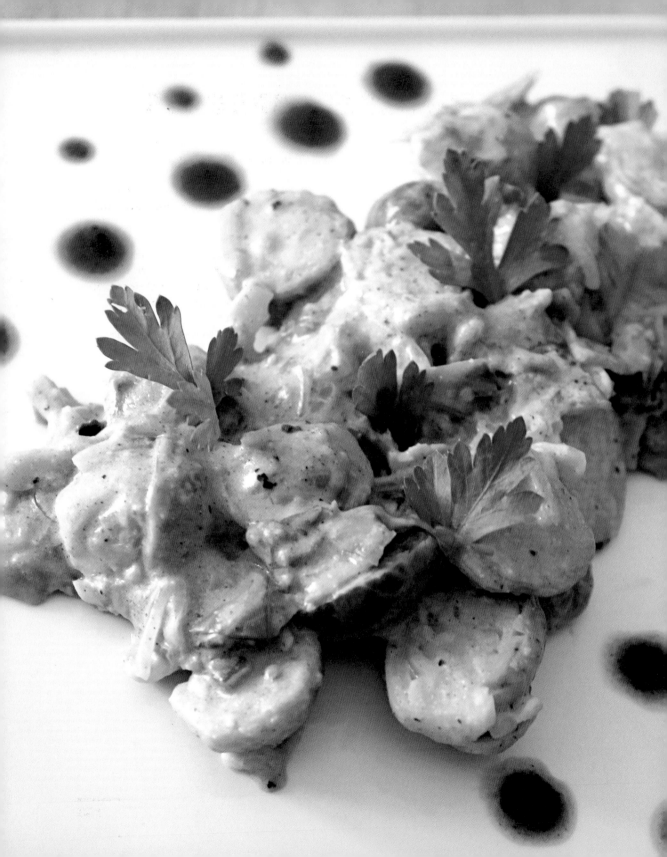

DREAMY BRUSSELS SPROUTS

You either love them or you hate them—Brussels sprouts, that is. They get a bad reputation because they are rarely cooked right. And by that I mean, these aren't your mom's boiled-into-mush Brussels sprouts. When they're roasted, with that crispy outside, they can be divine. The flavorful creamy sauce they're coated with in this recipe doesn't hurt either.

MAKES 2 MEDIUM BOWLS OF SPROUTS

2 cups Brussels sprouts
1 tablespoon vegan margarine
¼ cup chopped Vidalia onion
¼ cup Coconut Sour Cream (page 18)
2 teaspoons stone-ground mustard
½ teaspoon kosher salt
1 tablespoon pure maple syrup
¼ teaspoon ground black pepper

1. Preheat the oven to 350 degrees F.

2. Trim the stems of the Brussels sprouts and any outer leaves. Wash them and then halve them lengthwise.

3. In an 8 x 8-inch baking dish, place the Brussels sprouts, vegan margarine, onion, Coconut Sour Cream, mustard, kosher salt, ground black pepper, and maple syrup. Toss until well coated.

4. Bake for 20 minutes, then let cool and serve.

This is a super-easy side to go with your Balsamic Garlic Portobello Chop (page 124). This Brussels sprout recipe is almost like creamed onions, but you can also just keep it simple and toss your Brussels sprouts with a little bit of vegan margarine and a little bit of maple syrup and throw them in a 350 degree F oven for 15 minutes. Either version is guaranteed to change any Brussels hater's mind.

GARLIC CAULIFLOWER MASH

I never want to mess with perfection, and mashed potatoes are just that. The feeling you get when you indulge in the creamy mixture of potato, butter, milk, and salt to make mashed potatoes is undeniable. It is not the healthiest for you, though, so I wanted to still be able to get that comfort without all the starch and saturated fats. Cauliflower, coconut oil, and almond milk make the perfect substitutions. Cauliflower can make all your mashed dreams come true. Get creative and add some fresh herbs you have around the kitchen as well.

MAKES 5 SERVINGS OR 2 CUPS OF MASH

1 large head of cauliflower, trimmed and chopped
1 tablespoon coconut oil
¼ cup unsweetened almond milk
4 cloves garlic, minced
1 tablespoon chopped fresh chives, plus more for
 garnish
Kosher salt and freshly ground black pepper to taste

1. In a large pot, bring salted water to a boil.

2. Add the cauliflower and cook until the florets are tender, about 10 minutes.

3. Drain the cauliflower, then transfer to a blender.

4. Add the coconut oil, almond milk, garlic, chives, and kosher salt and pepper to taste.

5. Pulse until smooth but not liquefied.

6. Plate and sprinkle more chives on top.

Top with vegan margarine if you would like. Although, this garlic cauliflower mash is creamy enough on its own.

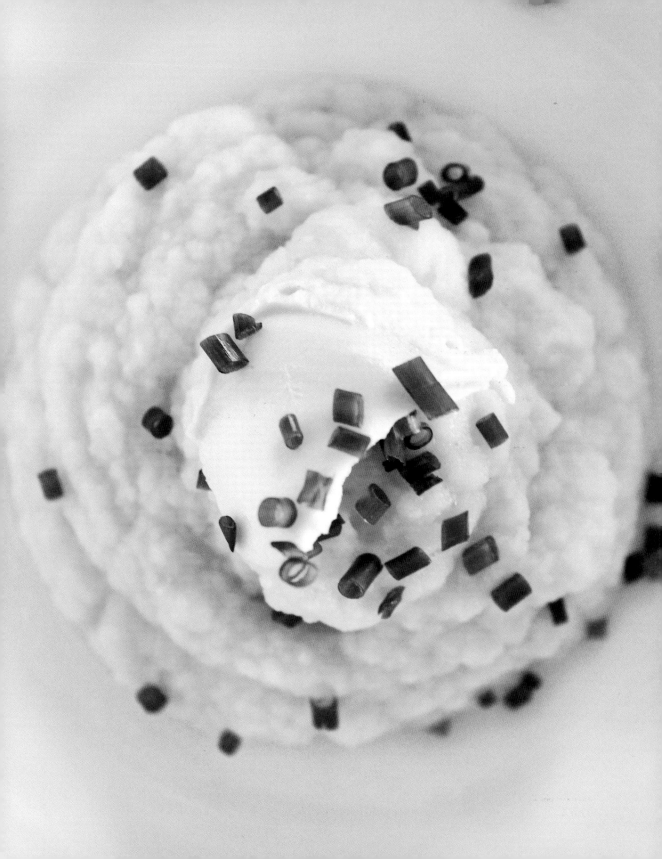

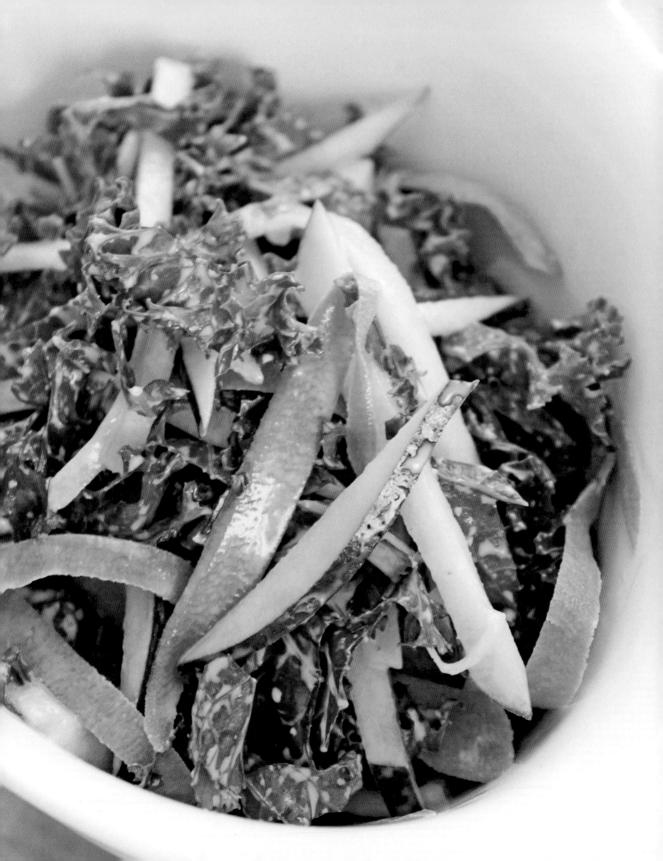

PEAR KALE SLAW

The first time I had a sweet slaw was in Houston, Texas. It was at a hole-in-the-wall joint downtown. They added apple to the napa cabbage, and I was completely blown away. I loved it so much that I asked for an extra container to take home. Mind you, it was only supposed to be put on the sandwiches. Regardless, it changed my mind about slaw forever because I realized that slaw didn't have to be just about cabbage. I started making it out of anything I could shred: beets, cucumbers, peppers, Brussels sprouts, onion, and even eggplant! That's when things got a little weird and I had to stop my obsession with slaw. In the end, I arrived at this perfectly harmonious slaw.

MAKES 4 SMALL PLATES OF SLAW

3 cups chopped kale leaves
3 pears, seeded and thinly sliced
1 large carrot, julienned
½ cup vegan mayonnaise
2 tablespoons organic apple cider vinegar
1 tablespoon pure maple syrup
½ teaspoon kosher salt
⅛ teaspoon freshly ground black pepper
1 bunch of scallions, thinly sliced
¼ cup minced fresh flat-leaf parsley

1. In a large bowl, toss the kale, pears, and carrot.

2. In a small bowl, mix the vegan mayonnaise, apple cider vinegar, maple syrup, kosher salt, pepper, scallions, and parsley.

3. Combine the mayo mixture with the kale, pears, and carrots and toss to coat.

4. Refrigerate for an hour and serve.

N This slaw is great as a side or served on sandwiches like the Shiitake Mushroom Po'Boy with Remoulade (page 104). Don't worry about massaging the kale—the mayo will break it down during refrigeration.

LUCY'S LICORICE (AKA PICKLED BEET STEMS)

I refused to eat beets as a kid, mostly because they were always doused in vinegar, and vinegar and I were the worst enemies growing up. Now I can't get enough of the stuff. I want to pickle everything, beet stems included. Sautéing them just isn't enough for me. These pickled wonders are perfect for putting on sandwiches, or you can enjoy them on their own when you're looking for something sweet but nutritious.

**MAKES ONE 16-OUNCE JAR
OF PICKLED BEET STEMS**

1 cup water
½ cup organic apple cider vinegar
½ cup organic granulated sugar
4 whole cloves
½ teaspoon ground cinnamon
⅛ teaspoon ground nutmeg
1 teaspoon kosher salt
2 bunches of beet stems,
    or as many as you can fit in the jar

1. In a medium saucepan, combine the water, vinegar, sugar, cloves, cinnamon, nutmeg, and kosher salt over medium heat.

2. Stir until the sugar is dissolved. Then raise the heat a tiny bit, add the beet stems, and simmer for 2 minutes.

3. Remove the beet stems and place them in a glass jar.

4. Pour the vinegar solution over the beets and let cool to room temperature.

5. Refrigerate until ready to eat. Keeps for up to 20 days.

You can mince the stems and put them over your favorite ice cream!

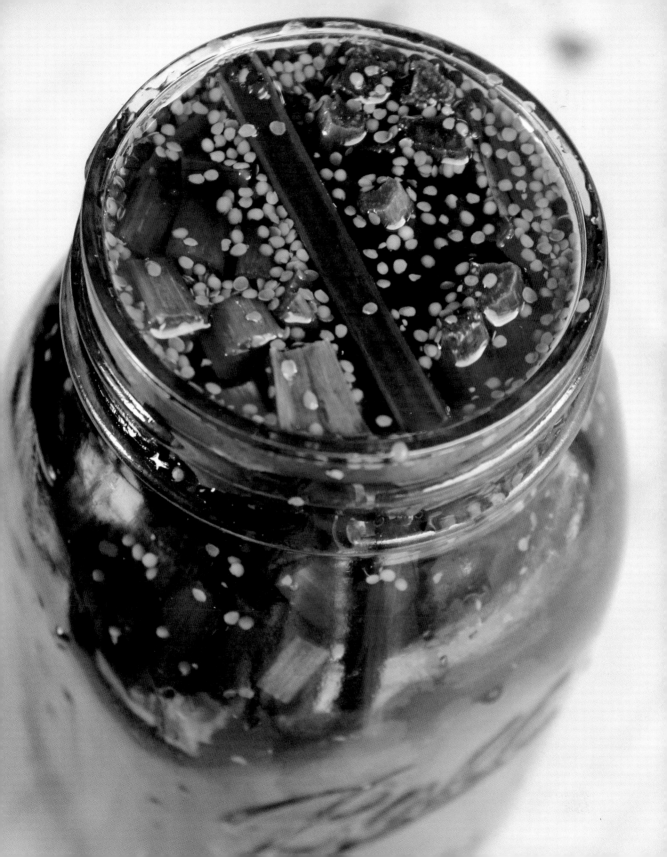

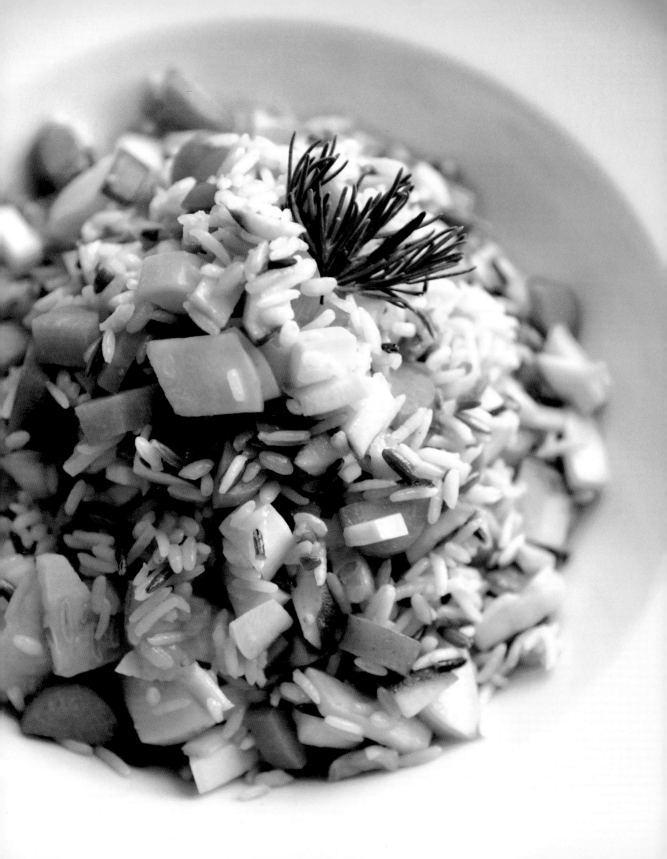

WILD RICE WITH CARROTS, ZUCCHINI, AND YELLOW SQUASH WITH GARLIC TRUFFLE BUTTER

There are many different varieties of rice you can find at the store nowadays. Wild rice is visually appealing as well as flavorful, and it goes great with fresh produce. For this recipe, I wanted a sauce that would really keep the natural flavor of the rice and vegetables but had a light, vibrant taste of its own. Truffle butter is the perfect sauce. To add more flavor, you can add whatever herbs you have lying around, such as rosemary, parsley, or basil.

MAKES 4 SMALL PLATES

2 cups Vegetable Broth (page 19)
1 cup wild rice
⅔ cup vegan butter
1 teaspoon black truffle oil
1 teaspoon garlic powder
2 carrots, diced
2 zucchini, diced
2 yellow squash, diced
Pinch of kosher salt

 Can't find wild rice? Use a rice that you have in the cupboard or pick one up that you've never cooked before.

1. In a large skillet, bring the vegetable broth to a boil over high heat.

2. Add the wild rice and cover the skillet with a lid.

3. Reduce the heat to medium-low and simmer for about 16 minutes, or until the rice has absorbed the broth.

4. While the rice is cooking, start on the garlic truffle butter. Place the vegan butter, black truffle oil, and garlic powder in a medium saucepan over medium heat. Cook until the butter is melted.

5. Remove the garlic truffle butter from the stove and cool.

6. Once the rice is ready, add the carrots, zucchini, and squash and toss. Cover and let sit for 5 to 7 minutes, until all the liquid is dissolved.

7. Pour the garlic truffle butter over the wild rice and vegetables. Add a pinch of salt, toss until well combined, and serve.

ROASTED GARLIC PARM CARROTS

It is no secret that I love garlic. It's always best to stay a safe distance away while having a conversation with me, especially if I've recently made these garlic-heavy crispy carrots. This strikingly beautiful dish brings color to a plate. And best of all, it gives you time to do whatever it is you want to do before dinner. It's the least time-consuming side dish I can think of. Remember to wash the carrots before you cook them, and don't peel them. The skin will give the carrots a nice texture when they roast.

MAKES 4 SERVINGS

8 large thin carrots (if they're thick, just cut in half vertically), unpeeled
1 tablespoon pure maple syrup
2 tablespoons coconut oil
1 teaspoon garlic powder
½ teaspoon onion powder
2 tablespoons chopped fresh flat-leaf parsley
¼ cup finely chopped cashews
1 tablespoon nutritional yeast
¼ teaspoon sea salt

1. Preheat the oven to 400 degrees F.

2. Place the carrots, maple syrup, coconut oil, garlic powder, onion powder, and parsley in a 9 x 13-inch baking dish. Mix to coat.

3. Bake for 20 minutes or until just brown.

4. Place on a serving dish and sprinkle with cashews, nutritional yeast, and sea salt.

N These carrots are deliciously creamy on the inside and slightly crispy on the outside. They are my favorite side to serve with pretty much any dish and great as a main course for lunch as well. Just serve them with some fresh raw spinach, raisins, and your favorite dressing!

DRUNKEN POTATOES

During a cooking class I once hosted we were drinking some ale, and somehow we came up with the idea to try to incorporate it into the potato side dish I was demonstrating. I'd never cooked with ale before, so I was skeptical. It could be that the ale helped me try it! In the end, these creamy potatoes were just right with the extra added kick of the hops.

MAKES 4 SMALL PLATES OF POTATOES

¼ cup vegan margarine
½ cup unsweetened almond milk
12 ounce vegan amber ale
3 medium shallots, sliced
½ cup nutritional yeast
1 teaspoon garlic powder
2 tablespoons chopped fresh flat-leaf parsley
½ teaspoon sea salt
¼ teaspoon freshly ground black pepper
2 pounds red potatoes, scrubbed and chopped

1. In a large skillet, heat the vegan margarine and the almond milk over medium-high heat. Bring to a boil.

2. Add the ale, shallots, nutritional yeast, garlic powder, parsley, sea salt, and pepper.

3. Reduce the heat to medium and add the potatoes.

4. Cover the pot and let simmer for 20 minutes or until all the liquid has evaporated.

Sprinkle whatever fresh herbs you have on top and garnish with a lemon wedge. This is a great side for Southern Fried Buttermilk Tofu (page 145).

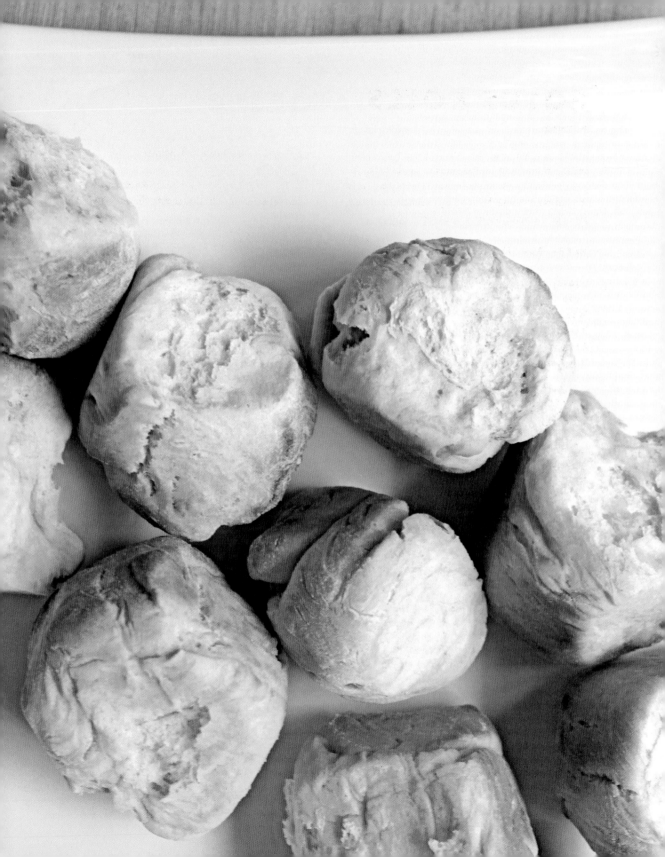

ROYCE ROLLS

Dinner rolls will always be a staple in my house. The smell of them baking and the wicker basket I usually put them in when I take them to the table will always remind me of home. These rolls are simple to make, even for the most beginner of bakers.

MAKES ABOUT 12 ROLLS

1 packet fast-acting dry yeast
1 cup warm water
¼ cup organic granulated sugar
3 cups sifted unbleached all-purpose flour
2 teaspoons sea salt
Vegan margarine, to grease baking pan

 These are delicious with Maple Cinnamon Butter. To make the butter, mix 3 tablespoons vegan margarine, 2 tablespoons maple syrup, and 1 teaspoon cinnamon. You can also make a more savory spread by using whatever spices and fresh herbs you have to make your own butter. Chopped rosemary, thyme, and parsley make a for a great savory butter. Get creative.

1. Preheat the oven to 400 degrees F.

2. In a large bowl, mix the yeast, water, and sugar and set aside until frothy, about 10 minutes.

3. Slowly add the flour and sea salt and mix until the dough is firm and slightly sticky.

4. Cover the bowl with a damp towel and let sit at room temperature.

5. Allow the dough to double in size. This will take 30 to 45 minutes.

6. Grease an 8 x 8-inch baking pan.

7. Once the dough has doubled in size, place it on a floured surface. Roll it out into a rope about 1 foot long. Cut the dough into 12 pieces. Place each piece neatly in the greased baking pan. You can crowd them; when baked, they will pull apart.

8. Bake for 20 minutes, until the tops are golden brown.

CILANTRO CHILI LIME BUTTER CORN

Fresh corn is a perfect taste on its own. But put this Cilantro Chili Lime Butter on it and your mind will be blown by the flavor. It has a deep, sweet, and earthy taste, with a nice spicy kick. Although some people say cilantro tastes like soap to them, I think it tastes like summer. Feel free to substitute the cilantro with your favorite fresh herb.

MAKES 4 EARS OF CORN

¼ cup vegan margarine
½ tablespoon freshly squeezed lime juice
2 tablespoons chili sauce, plus move for serving
¼ teaspoon kosher salt
¼ teaspoon freshly ground black pepper
4 ears of corn
¼ cup chopped fresh cilantro

1. Preheat the oven to 400 degrees F.

2. In a small bowl, mix together the vegan margarine, lime juice, chili sauce, kosher salt, and pepper.

3. Rub the chili-lime mix on all the corn ears until lightly coated.

4. Wrap each corn individually in foil.

5. Place the ears of corn directly on the oven racks and bake for 20 minutes.

6. Unwrap the foil and let the corn cool for 5 minutes.

7. Cut each ear of corn in half and sprinkle with cilantro and more chili sauce, if desired.

N You can spice up your corn a number of different ways. Mix your favorite spices—chili powder, cumin, paprika, etc.—with some vegan butter and you've got yourself a new side dish.

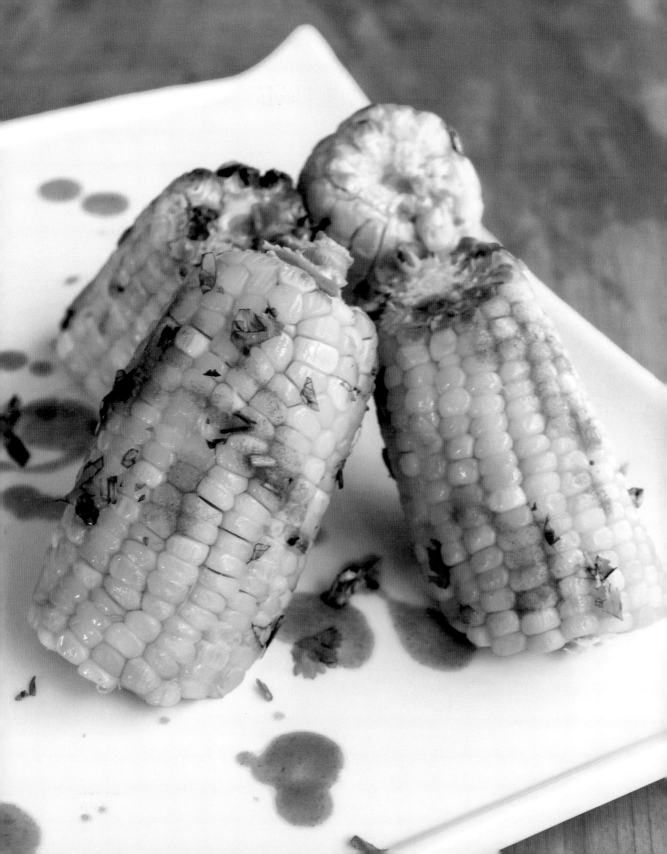

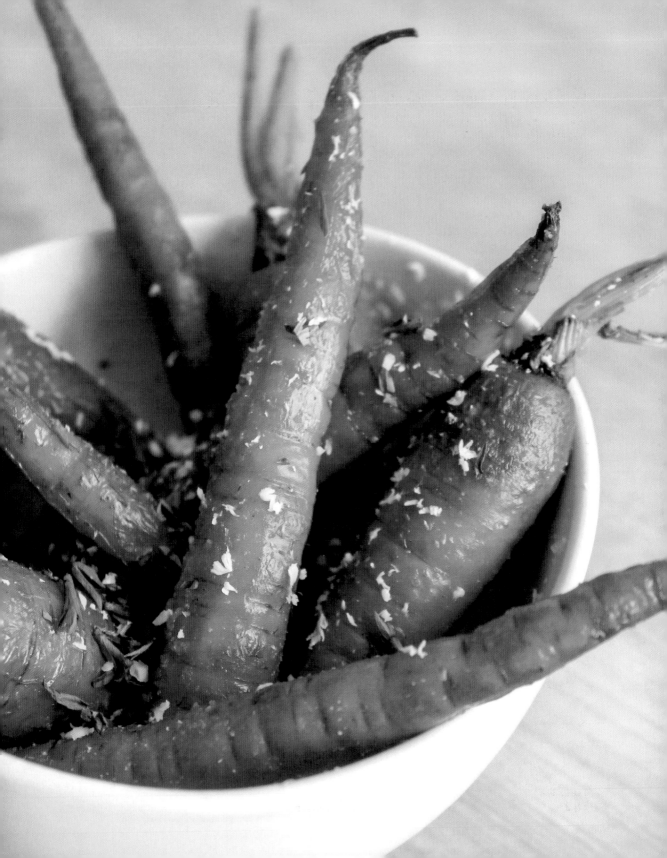

ROSEMARY OLIVE OIL BISCUIT MUFFINS

Sometimes you just can't decide between two foods, and when that happens you just have to combine them. Indecision was my inspiration for these Rosemary Olive Oil Biscuit Muffins. I wanted to make a breakfast muffin, but I also wanted something a little lighter and a lot more yeasty, like a biscuit. Baking these in a muffin tin gives them a perfect crisp without making them as dense and as hard as a rock. And who doesn't love rosemary and olive oil together? These muffins are great for a lunchtime snack or perfect for a dinner side.

MAKES 12 MUFFINS

1 packet highly active yeast
¼ cup water
2 tablespoons organic granulated sugar
2½ cups sifted unbleached all-purpose flour
1 teaspoon baking powder
2 tablespoons fresh rosemary, chopped
1 teaspoon kosher salt
½ cup extra-virgin olive oil
1 cup unsweetened almond milk
1 tablespoon organic apple cider vinegar
Coconut oil cooking spray or flour, to prep
    the muffin tin

1. In a small bowl, mix the yeast, water, and sugar.

2. In a large bowl, mix the flour, baking powder, rosemary, kosher salt, and olive oil.

3. In another small bowl, mix the almond milk and apple cider vinegar and let sit until the milk starts to curdle.

4. Add the yeast and almond milk mixture to the flour and mix until a sticky dough forms.

5. Cover the bowl with a damp towel and let it rise for 1 hour.

6. Preheat the oven to 400 degrees F.

7. Pat the dough down and scrape it away from the sides of the bowl to make it easier to remove.

8. Grease a muffin tin with coconut oil cooking spray or simply dust with flour.

9. Using a spoon, fill each muffin cup two-thirds of the way up.

10. Bake for 10 minutes or until the muffin tops are golden brown.

 Serve these hot with some vegan margarine.

MAPLE TEMPEH BACON

Bacon culture is a huge phenomenon, and I totally understand why. The smoky saltiness of bacon is worthy of obsession. Since I have a love for all things sweet and salty, I added some maple to make this tempeh bacon just right. The maple also helps give the tempeh bacon a crispy outside coating when you pan-fry them.

MAKES 12 STRIPS OF TEMPEH BACON

1 (8-ounce) package tempeh bacon
¼ cup pure maple syrup
1 tablespoon soy sauce
1 teaspoon liquid smoke
¼ cup organic apple cider vinegar
½ teaspoon ground cumin
1 teaspoon freshly ground black pepper
Pinch of sea salt

1. Cut the tempeh into 6 pieces to make long strips. Then cut those pieces in half, leaving you with 12 strips.

2. In a deep baking dish, mix the maple syrup, soy sauce, liquid smoke, apple cider vinegar, cumin, pepper, and sea salt.

3. Add the tempeh bacon and toss to coat.

4. Let the tempeh bacon marinate for 30 minutes.

5. Heat a large cast-iron skillet over medium-high heat. (Don't worry if you don't have a cast-iron skillet; use the skillet you have.) Place the tempeh bacon strips in the skillet and cook for 4 minutes, then flip the strips and cook for 4 minutes more. There should be a crust that forms a crispy layer on the outside of the tempeh.

Never heard of liquid smoke before? Don't stress—neither had I, until I wanted to try to turn every vegetable into bacon. You can find it in your local grocery store in the same aisle as barbecue sauce and hot sauce.

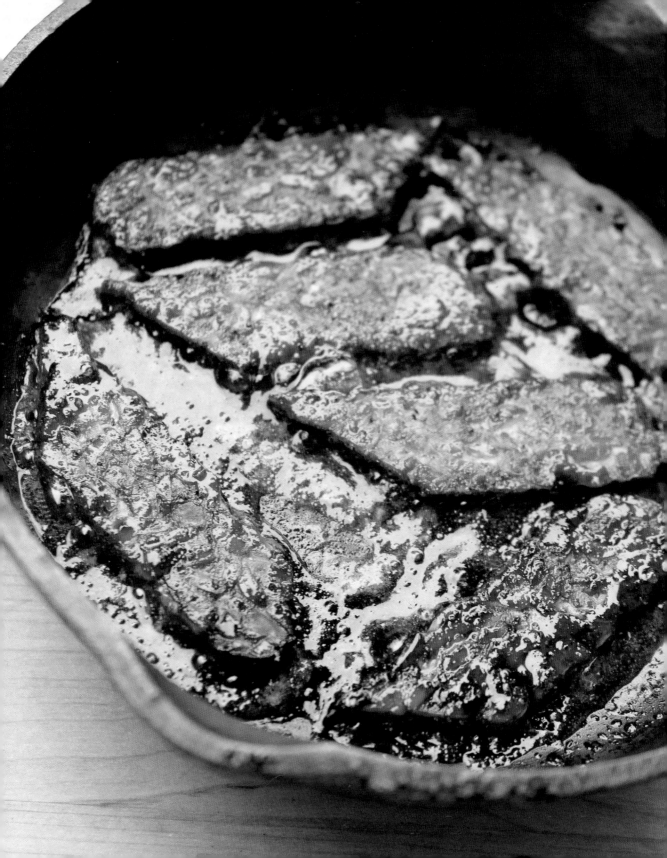

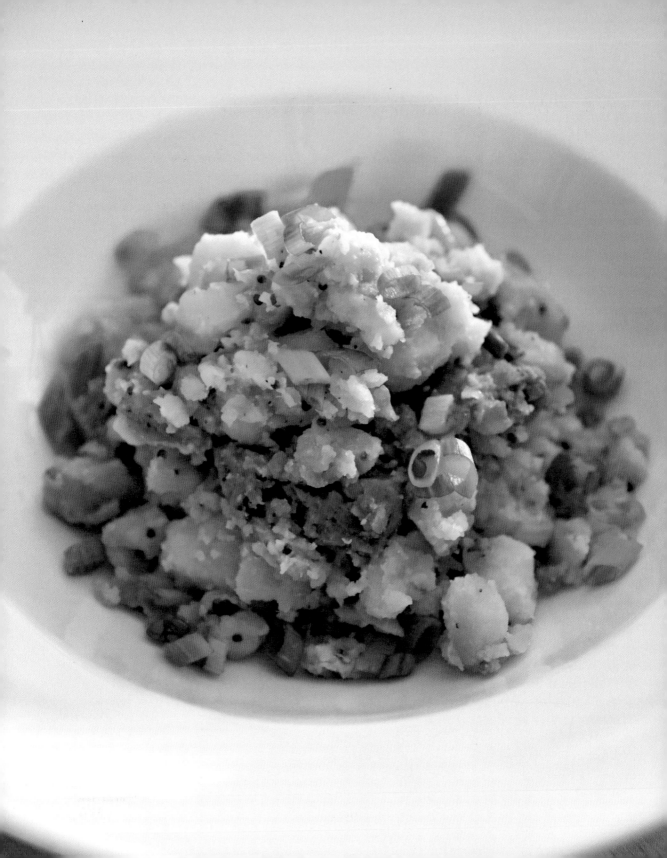

GERMAN POTATO SALAD

A while before I went vegan, I dated a guy who was. This was way before there were any vegan alternatives, and it was my first real glimpse into what veganism was. Back then I didn't know how to cook, so I took to the Internet to show me some food I could bring—that wasn't just a salad or vegan cookies—to a barbecue he was having. I chose German potato salad and it was a huge hit. Years later, I got in the kitchen and decided to make my own version.

MAKES 5 SERVINGS

1 pound Yukon Gold potatoes, scrubbed and chopped
1 pound red potatoes, scrubbed and chopped
⅓ cup white vinegar
2 tablespoons coconut oil
½ cup capers
¾ cup chopped yellow onion
¼ cup (packed) organic brown sugar
1 tablespoon stone-ground mustard
¼ cup chopped scallion greens
Salt and freshly ground black pepper to taste

1. Bring a large pot of salted water and the potatoes to a boil over high heat.

2. Cook the potatoes for 10 to 15 minutes, until soft.

3. Drain the potatoes and set aside in a large bowl.

4. In a large saucepan, whisk the vinegar and coconut oil over low heat.

5. Add the capers, onion, brown sugar, and mustard.

6. Add the cooked potatoes. Toss to coat and remove from the heat.

7. Add the scallions and salt and pepper to taste.

 If you have Maple Tempeh Bacon (page 170) lying around, throw some in for a twist on this German dish.

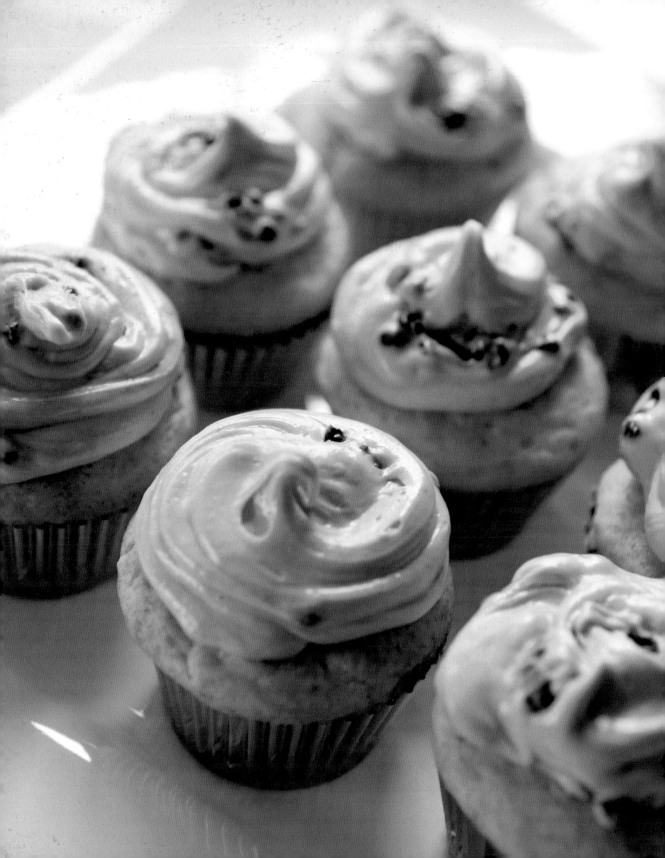

DESSERTS

Baking was never my thing growing up. But when I started eating a plant-based diet, I learned how satisfying baking (especially without dairy) could really be. Ironically, it was after I made the best and healthiest lifestyle change of my life—becoming vegan—that I developed a voracious sweet tooth. Call me crazy, but I really think that vegan desserts can be just as good as, if not better than, dairy desserts.

Beginner vegans are often afraid that they'll have to give up their favorite snacks and treats, and I'm happy to tell you that that is simply not the case. In this chapter you'll find everything from American Apple Pie to Double Trouble Brownies. We're covering all those delicious comfort food bases. So get baking!

AMERICAN APPLE PIE

This is by far my favorite dessert. Put a scoop of vanilla coconut ice cream on top and you are good to go. My grandmother taught me to use thick apples growing up, but I prefer to use thinly sliced apples. It gives you a lighter and more tart-like pie.

MAKES 8 PIECES OF PIE

CRUST
1½ cups sifted unbleached all-purpose flour, plus more to dust the pie tin
½ teaspoon sea salt
½ cup vegan margarine
¼ cup ice cold water

PIE FILLING
5 apples of your choice, cored, peeled, and thinly sliced
Freshly squeezed juice of ½ medium lemon
1½ tablespoons ground cinnamon
½ cup (packed) organic light brown sugar

 When you are cutting the apples, squeeze the lemon juice over them in the bowl to keep them from browning.

Serve with vanilla coconut ice cream and garnish with fresh mint.

1. Preheat the oven to 350 degrees F.

2. To make the crust: In a medium bowl, mix the flour and sea salt together.

3. Add the vegan margarine and mix by hand until the mixture forms into big crumbles.

4. Add the water one tablespoon at a time until the pie dough is firm.

5. Roll the dough into a ball and place it in plastic wrap. Refrigerate for 1 hour.

6. To make the pie filling: In a large bowl, mix the apples, lemon juice, cinnamon, and brown sugar.

7. Dust a 9-inch pie tin with flour. This will keep the bottom and sides of the crust from sticking. Do not use margarine to grease the tin (it will give you a soft bottom crust).

8. Place the piecrust in the center of the pie tin and push to form the shape of the pie tin. Press the dough evenly so the piecrust is a uniform thickness. You can roll it out as well, but I just find shaping it less time-consuming. Cut away any excess dough.

9. Place the apple mixture in the piecrust and spread it evenly.

10. Bake for 40 to 50 minutes. Keep an eye on it after 40 minutes to make sure the crust isn't burning.

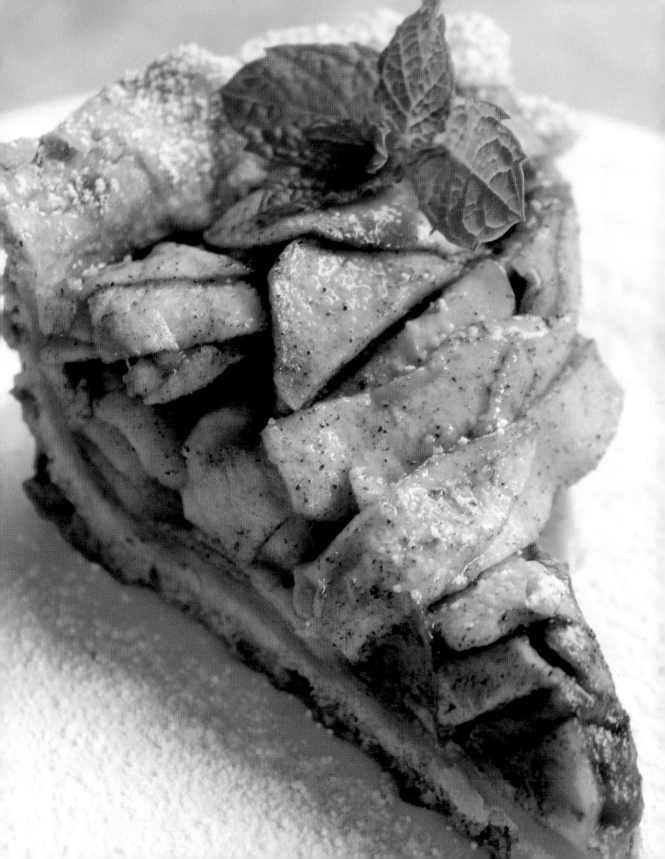

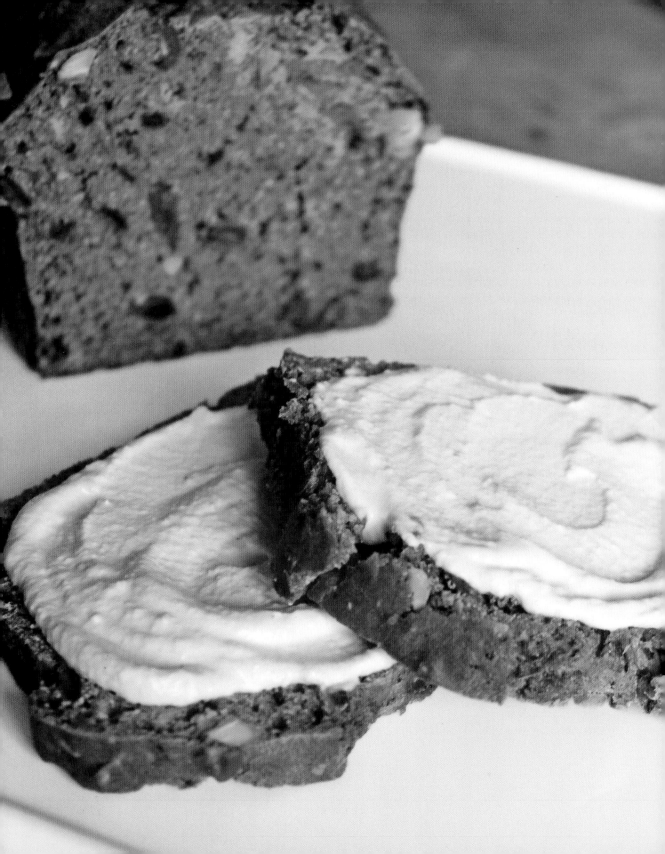

GRANDMA MATTERN'S DATE NUT BREAD

My dad's mother, whom I was named after, is the inspiration for this recipe. I can't say she was a woman who had a very diverse palate, but she was still a woman with taste. She knew what she liked and exactly how she liked it. Date nut bread is a good example—it was a huge staple in her household. If we went to her house before noon, it was almost inevitable that she'd make us eat it with cream cheese. I say "make" because I absolutely did not do it willingly, mostly because I thought dates were the same as prunes, and as a kid the "prune" word is horrifying. Now I've grown to love dates and this bread. Mary Mattern is the reason I'll always cherish recipe writing, because although she's not with us anymore, she will always be in my kitchen—and yours, too, when you make this recipe.

MAKES 10 SLICES OF BREAD

1 cup dates, pitted and chopped
1 cup boiling water
2 cups sifted unbleached all-purpose flour
1 tablespoon baking powder
1 teaspoon baking soda
½ teaspoon sea salt
½ teaspoon ground cinnamon
¼ teaspoon ground allspice
1 tablespoon ground flaxseed meal
3 tablespoons water
2 tablespoons organic granulated sugar
1 tablespoon vegan margarine, melted
1 teaspoon pure vanilla extract
¼ cup pure maple syrup
¼ cup strong coffee
¼ cup chopped walnuts
¼ cup chopped pecans

1. Preheat the oven to 350 degrees F.

2. Grease a 9 x 5 x 3-inch loaf pan and set aside.

3. In a small bowl, combine the dates and boiling water and let cool.

4. In a large bowl, mix the flour, baking powder, baking soda, sea salt, cinnamon, and allspice.

5. In another small bowl, mix the flaxseed meal and water. Let sit until the flaxseed meal absorbs the water.

6. Add the sugar, vegan margarine, and vanilla to the flaxseed meal mixture. Beat for 1 minute.

7. Pour the flaxseed mixture and dates (with water) into the flour mixture. Add the maple syrup, coffee, walnuts, and pecans. Mix until well combined.

8. Pour the mixture into the prepared bread pan and bake for 1 hour or until a toothpick inserted into the center of the loaf comes out clean.

9. Let the bread cool to room temperature, then remove from the loaf pan and slice.

GRANDMA BENSON'S BLUEBERRY CAKE

I never got the chance to meet my mom's mom, since she passed away before I was born. Among the amazing stories I've heard about her are tales about this blueberry cake. My mom tells me they ate it every Sunday in the summer. She actually found the original recipe my grandmother wrote and sent it out in an e-mail to the whole family. I was excited to have a piece of her in the kitchen with me, but as soon as I looked at the ingredients, I knew it was going to be a bit of a challenge to change the recipe to suit my needs; it was laden with eggs and milk, like many great cake recipes. But I was determined to celebrate my grandmother's legacy and create a plant-based version of her cake that she would be proud of. I think you'll agree that it's absolutely delicious!

MAKES 12 SLICES OF CAKE

¼ cup vegan margarine
¾ cup organic granulated sugar
1 tablespoon flaxseed meal
3 tablespoons water
1¼ cups sifted unbleached all-purpose flour, plus
    ½ cup more for flouring
1½ teaspoons baking powder
½ cup unsweetened almond milk
¼ teaspoon sea salt
2 cups fresh blueberries, rinsed and patted dry

1. Preheat the oven to 350 degrees F.

2. In a large bowl, mix the vegan margarine and sugar until creamed.

3. In a small bowl, mix the flaxseed meal and water. Let the mixture sit until the flaxseed meal absorbs most of the water.

4. Add the flaxseed meal to the vegan margarine and sugar mixture.

5. Add 1¼ cups of the sifted flour, baking powder, almond milk, and sea salt.

6. In medium bowl, toss the blueberries in the remaining ½ cup flour until lightly coated.

7. Place the blueberries in the cake mixture. Discard any extra flour left over from flouring the blueberries.

8. Gently fold the blueberries into the batter.

9. Pour the batter into a greased 8 x 8-inch pan.

10. Bake for 45 to 50 minutes, or until the center of the cake is done. You can test this by inserting a toothpick into the center of the cake. If it comes out clean, your cake is ready! If it does not, keep it in for a couple minutes longer.

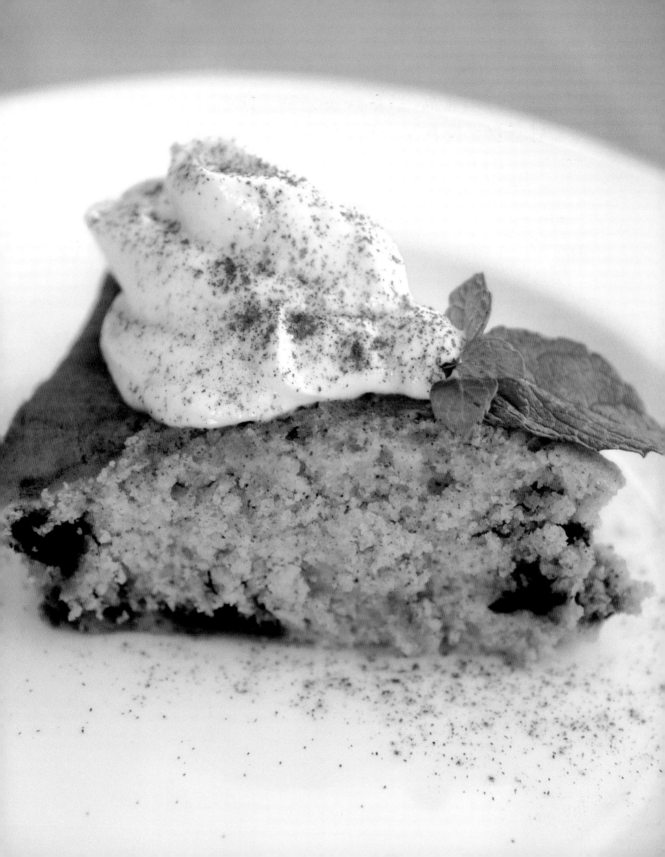

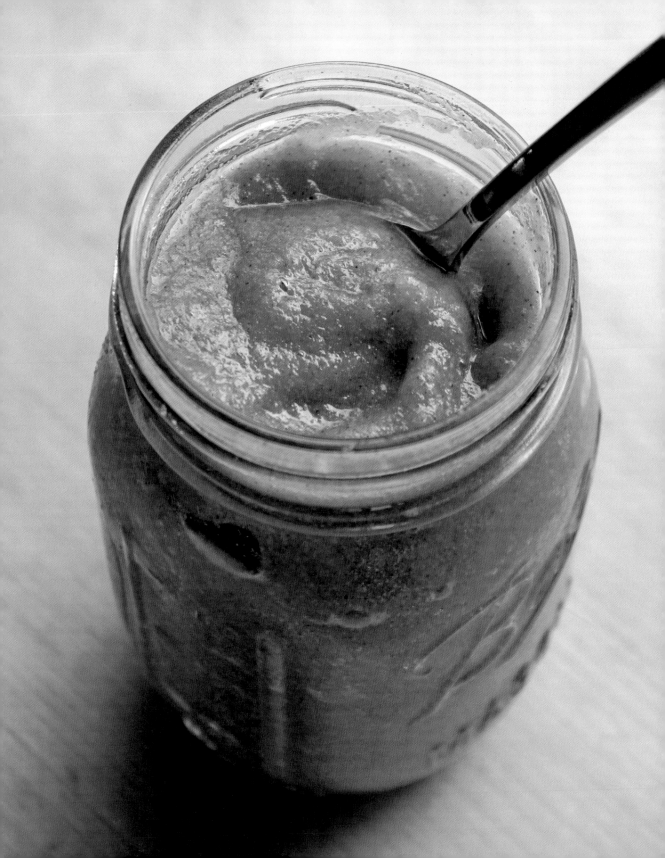

RAW CINNAMON APPLESAUCE

I think I legitimately thought applesauce cured every sickness when I was younger. Common cold? Applesauce. Chicken pox? Applesauce. Fell out of a tree? Applesauce. Which is why I was sick of it by age sixteen, when I became too cool for anything that even resembled baby food. Then one day I had way too many apples left over from apple picking. I decided that I'd spend all day making applesauce in the kitchen. A half hour later, I was done and the kitchen was clean. I sat and ate applesauce for the rest of the day. That's the moment I realized that healthy and delicious food does not have to be complicated and that you are never too old for comforting "kid" food.

MAKES 2 CUPS OF APPLESAUCE

6 apples, peeled, cored, and chopped
5 dates, pitted and chopped
½ tablespoon ground cinnamon
1 tablespoon freshly squeezed lemon juice

1. Place the apples, dates, cinnamon, and lemon juice in the bowl of a blender and blend until smooth.

2. Eat right away or store in a glass jar. Keeps for up to 30 days.

N Aside from picking up fresh fruit and putting it straight into your mouth, this is by far the easiest fruit snack or dish to make, especially when you have no time. You can even substitute pears for the apples and make pear sauce.

FAT MINT CHIP COOKIES

Sometimes I think the meaning of life really is to just find the chocolate chip cookie recipe you love most. There are so many different ways to make a chocolate chip cookie, and it all comes down to preference. Chewy? Soft? Crunchy? Cakey? I like mine to be a balance of all those descriptors. Oh, and almost always with mint.

MAKES 12 COOKIES

¾ cup vegan margarine
1⅓ cups organic granulated sugar
1 tablespoon pure vanilla extract
1 teaspoon mint extract
1 tablespoon ground flaxseed meal
3 tablespoons warm water
2 cups sifted unbleached all-purpose flour
½ teaspoon sea salt
½ teaspoon baking soda
½ teaspoon cream of tartar
1 (16-ounce) bag vegan chocolate chips

1. Preheat the oven to 350 degrees F.

2. In a large bowl, mix the vegan margarine, sugar, vanilla, and mint extract.

3. In a small cup, mix the flaxseed meal and warm water. Then pour into the sugar mixture.

4. In another bowl, whisk the flour, sea salt, baking soda, and cream of tartar until combined.

5. Slowly mix the sugar mixture into the flour mixture until smooth.

6. Fold in the chocolate chips.

7. Place parchment paper on a cookie sheet.

8. Place a tablespoon of cookie dough on the cookie sheet. Repeat until all the dough is gone, leaving 1 inch between cookies.

9. Bake for 7 minutes. Use a metal spatula to transfer the cookies to a cooling rack. Let the cookies cool for about 15 minutes, then enjoy.

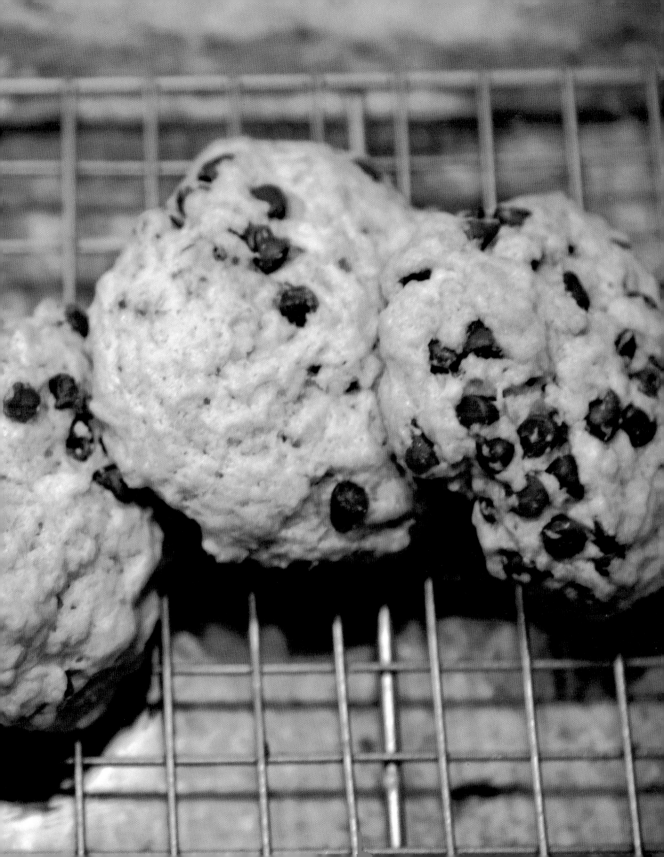

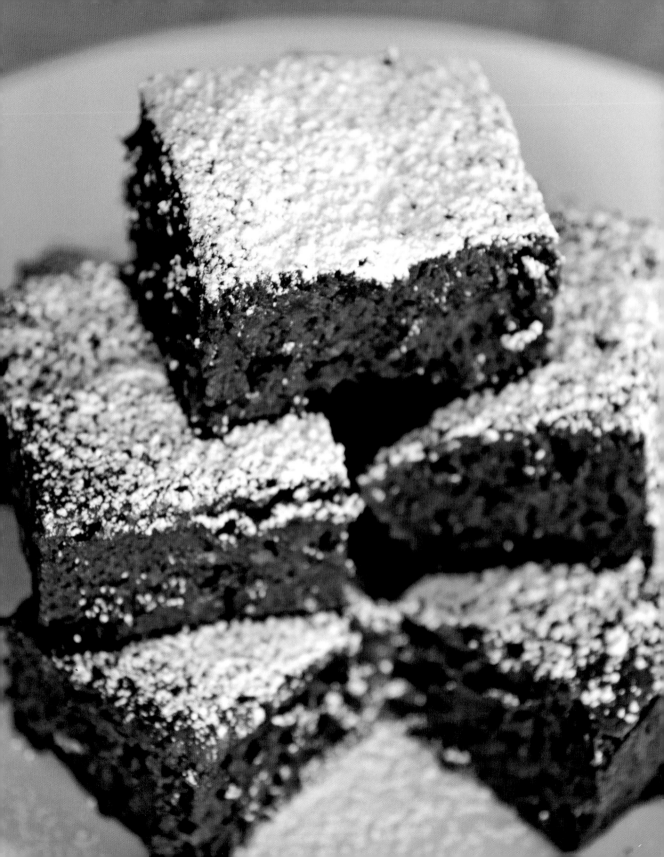

DOUBLE TROUBLE BROWNIES

For a very long time, any vegan brownie I made really came out more like cake. It was hard for me to let thick batter go into the oven. I was nervous that it wouldn't bake well, and I couldn't fight the urge to thin the batter out. Once I was able to hold myself back, I found the perfect consistency. Then I worked on shoving as much chocolate into the batter as possible. The result? These heavenly treats with their perfectly crisp tops and gooey centers. The chocolate chips give them a double burst of chocolate flavor. Also, no eggs = no salmonella. LICK THE BATTER!

MAKES 10 BROWNIES

Coconut oil cooking spray, to grease the baking pan
2 tablespoons ground flaxseed meal
3 tablespoons warm water
1 cup sifted unbleached all-purpose flour
½ cup cacao powder
¼ teaspoon baking powder
1 teaspoon sea salt
½ cup vegan margarine
¼ cup pure maple syrup
¼ cup unsweetened almond milk
2 teaspoons pure vanilla extract
1 cup vegan chocolate chips
Organic confectioners' sugar (optional)

1. Preheat the oven to 350 degrees F and grease a 9-inch square baking pan with coconut oil cooking spray.

2. In a small bowl, mix the flaxseed meal and water. Set aside.

3. In a large bowl, mix the flour, cacao powder, baking powder, and sea salt.

4. In a medium bowl, mix together the vegan margarine, maple syrup, almond milk, and vanilla.

5. Pour the flaxseed mixture and the margarine mixture into the flour mixture and mix until well combined.

6. Pour the batter into the prepared baking pan and bake for 30 minutes or until a toothpick inserted in the middle comes out clean.

7. Let the brownies cool for about an hour before serving.

8. Sprinkle with confectioners' sugar, if desired, and enjoy!

CITRUS CHOCOLATE MOUSSE

If you are not familiar with making chocolate mousse from avocados, you will likely think I'm a crazy person and flip to the next page. Plant-based chefs have been doing it for years. It's the healthiest substitute for dairy products and doesn't give up any of the taste. The creamy texture is pure decadence. What's more, it's also much, much easier to prepare than a traditional version.

MAKES 2 CUPS OF MOUSSE

3 ripe avocados, pitted, peeled, and chopped
¼ cup cacao powder
½ cup unsweetened almond milk
¼ cup freshly squeezed orange juice
¼ cup pure maple syrup
1½ teaspoons pure vanilla extract
Dash of sea salt
1 orange, sliced

1. In the bowl of a blender, add the avocados, cacao powder, almond milk, orange juice, maple syrup, vanilla, and sea salt. Blend until smooth.

2. Serve with fresh orange slices.

N Make sure the avocados you use are ripe. If they are not, you will end up with a chunky pudding. It will be no less delicious, but it will not have the smooth texture that you're looking for in a mousse.

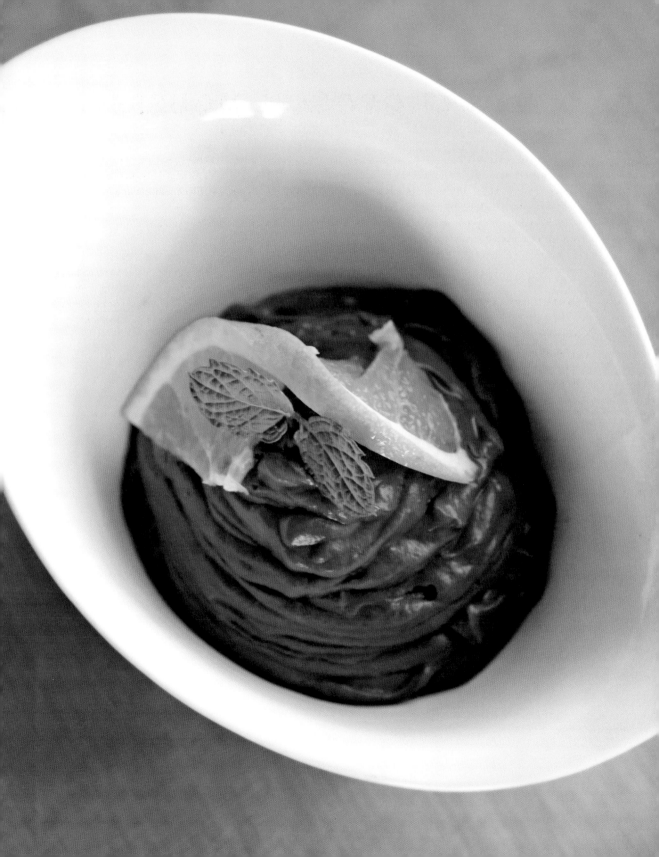

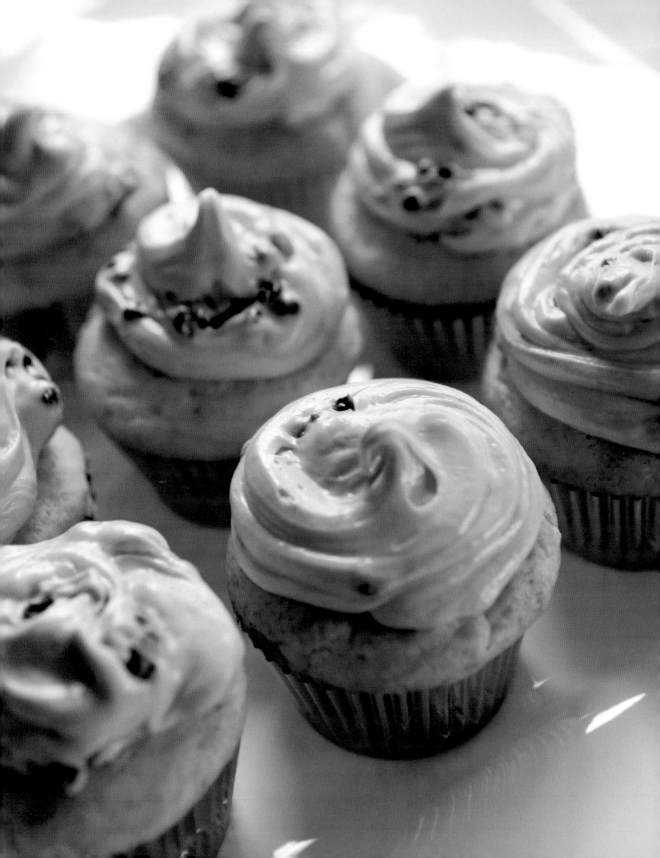

WHISKEY LADY CUPCAKES

My fondest memory of a fun time my sister and I had together was when we took a road trip and visited whiskey distilleries in Kentucky. For one of her recent birthdays, I decided to create a cupcake inspired by that adventure and by her love of the spirit. Whiskey makes a fine addition to your sweets.

MAKES 12 CUPCAKES

CUPCAKES
2⅓ cups sifted unbleached all-purpose flour
2 teaspoons baking powder
½ teaspoon baking soda
½ teaspoon cream of tartar
¼ teaspoon kosher salt
½ cup vegetable oil
1 cup organic granulated sugar
1½ cups unsweetened almond milk
1 tablespoon freshly squeezed lemon juice
1 teaspoon organic apple cider vinegar
2 teaspoons pure vanilla extract

FROSTING
½ cup vegan margarine
½ teaspoon bourbon whiskey
5 cups organic confectioners' sugar
3 tablespoons unsweetened almond milk
1½ teaspoons pure vanilla extract
Pinch of salt
½ cup raspberries

 This may seem like a lot of steps and ingredients, but it goes quickly, I promise. You'll be licking icing from the bowl in no time.

1. Preheat the oven to 350 degrees F.

2. To make the cupcakes: In a large bowl, mix together the flour, baking powder, baking soda, cream of tartar, and kosher salt.

3. In a small bowl, mix together the vegetable oil and sugar.

4. Pour the sugar mixture into the flour mixture.

5. Add the almond milk, lemon juice, apple cider vinegar, and vanilla and mix until smooth.

6. Place cupcake liners in cupcake tins and pour the batter one-third high in each liner. You can pour them two-thirds high if you like to have a cupcake top, but this will yield fewer cupcakes.

7. Bake for about 20 minutes. Keep an eye on them. Once the top is golden brown, place a toothpick in the center. If it comes out clean, they're ready!

8. Let the cupcakes cool in the cupcake tin for 15 minutes.

9. To make the frosting: In a large bowl, mix together the vegan margarine, bourbon, confectioners' sugar, almond milk, vanilla, and salt.

10. In a blender, blend the raspberries until smooth.

(CONTINUED)

11. In a fine-mesh strainer placed over a bowl, rub the raspberry puree and press out the juice.

12. Then strain through a cheesecloth to ensure there are not big chunks of raspberry left. Add the raspberry juice to the frosting mixture.

13. Place the frosting mixture in a pastry bag, a little at a time. Then pipe the frosting on top of cupcakes. If you don't have a pastry bag, you can always cut the corners of a large sandwich/freezer bag and either pipe the frosting straight from the bag or attach a tip and coupling.

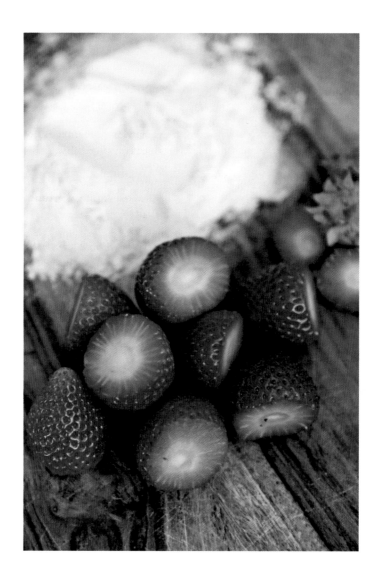

COCONUT-BATTERED STRAWBERRY ZEPPOLE

If you've ever been to a fair or carnival, you know that bright marquee sign with the almost-blinding shining lightbulbs means deep-fried everything. From funnel cakes to deep-fried cookies to deep-fried butter, you name it, you can deep-fry it at a carnival. I've always preferred the simpler fried dough, zeppoles. They'd give them to you in a bag with more confectioners' sugar than you knew what to do with. You'd shake the bag up to coat the hot dough and when you opened it, a perfect, sweet puff of confectioners' sugar would appear. These nostalgic memories are the inspiration for this recipe, only now I've created a filled version, which takes the original to new heights! With their strawberry center, these zeppoles are even more magical.

MAKES ABOUT 24 ZEPPOLES

2 cups water
1 cup coconut milk
½ teaspoon sea salt
¼ cup organic granulated sugar
1 tablespoon ground cinnamon
3 cups sifted unbleached all-purpose flour
Peanut oil, for frying
3 cups fresh strawberries, stemmed
½ cup organic confectioners' sugar

1. In a medium bowl, mix the water, coconut milk, sea salt, granulated sugar, and cinnamon.

2. Add the flour and stir until the batter is smooth. Add more water if the batter is too thick.

3. Heat about an inch of oil in a heavy-bottomed pot over medium heat to 360 degrees F. Use a candy/deep fry thermometer.

4. Dip the strawberries in the batter and carefully place in the oil. Fry them until they are until golden brown.

5. Remove the strawberries from the oil using a slotted spoon.

6. Place on a plate lined with paper towels. Using a sieve, sprinkle confectioners' sugar over the zeppoles.

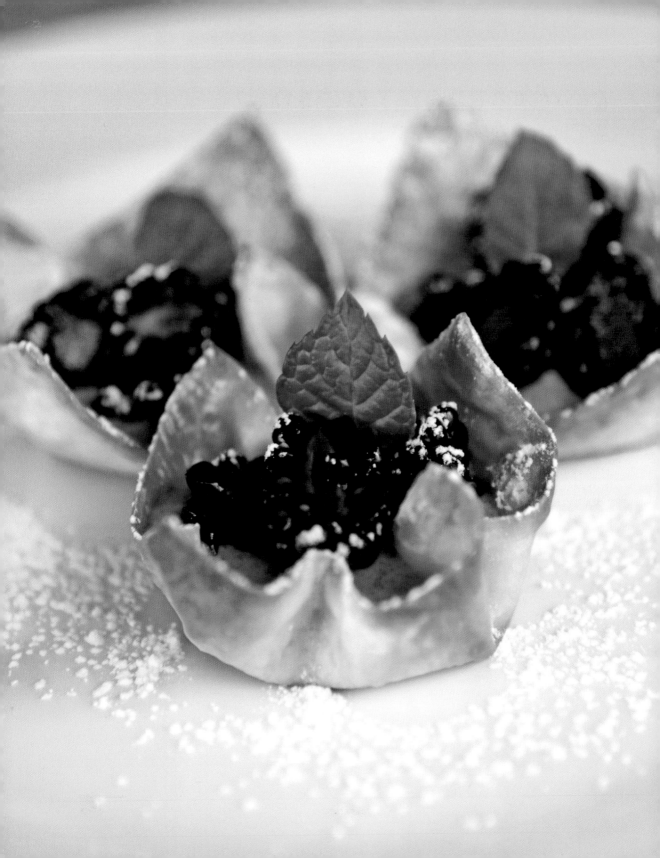

BLACKBERRY COCONUT WONTON CUPS

Blackberries are usually the loner berry. They get forgotten about a lot and are usually overshadowed by strawberries. But in this recipe, the blackberries are the star. You won't miss strawberries, or any other berries, one bit. The coconut balances out the tartness of the berries with its creamy sweetness, and the wontons give it the crunch you need to bring it all together. The shells are simple to make. It's the perfect last-minute dessert!

MAKES 20 WONTON CUPS

20 wonton wrappers

FILLING

3 (13.5-ounce) cans coconut cream, refrigerated
1 tablespoon ground cinnamon
1 cup chopped blackberries
1 cup confectioners' sugar, plus more to sprinkle on
  the wonton cups
1 bunch of fresh mint, for garnish

1. Preheat the oven to 375 degrees F.

2. Place a wonton wrapper over a muffin cup and push down with two fingers to make a cup within the tin.

3. Follow this until all the wonton wrappers are used. You will most likely need two or more muffin tins.

4. Bake for 5 to 6 minutes or until golden brown. Keep an eye on these, as they can burn easily.

5. To make the filling: In a small bowl, mix together the coconut milk fat, cinnamon, and confectioners' sugar. Make sure to only use the coconut cream from the can and not the liquid.

6. You can spoon the mixture into the cups or, to make them neat, use a piping bag or, realistically, a plastic sandwich bag.

7. Top with blackberries, sprinkle with confectioners' sugar through a fine-mesh strainer, and garnish with mint.

N I love this recipe with blackberries, but you can use blueberries or any other berries that are in season. You can even use peaches or mangoes, too.

DOUGHNUT HOLES

Some people think doughnut holes are a poor alternative to bigger and better whole doughnuts. I, on the other hand, think these bite-size dough balls are a wonder because they fry up perfectly crisp in every bite. They also allow us to portion out our desire for doughnuts a little bit more. Unless you eat all of them in one sitting (okay, maybe I have, too), in which case—forget I wrote that last sentence.

MAKES ABOUT 24 DOUGHNUTS

5 cups vegetable oil, for frying
1 cup unsweetened almond milk
1 tablespoon flaxseed meal
3 tablespoons water
2 cups sifted unbleached all-purpose flour
2 tablespoons organic granulated sugar
4½ teaspoons baking powder
½ teaspoon kosher salt
¼ cup vegan margarine, melted

1. Heat the oil to 350 degrees F in a heavy-bottomed pot. Use a candy/deep-fry thermometer.

2. In a large bowl, mix together the almond milk, flaxseed meal, water, flour, sugar, baking powder, kosher salt, and vegan margarine.

3. Scoop out the dough with a tablespoon, or use an ice cream scooper for a more circular shape.

4. Place the dough in the oil carefully and fry until golden brown, about 2 minutes.

5. Place on a tray lined with paper towels.

Nᴺ Roll these wonderful balls of fried goodness in cinnamon sugar or make a simple glaze such as the Autumn Glaze (page 33). If you want to get more creative, once the doughnut holes have cooled, poke a hole in the center and use a piping bag to squeeze jam inside.

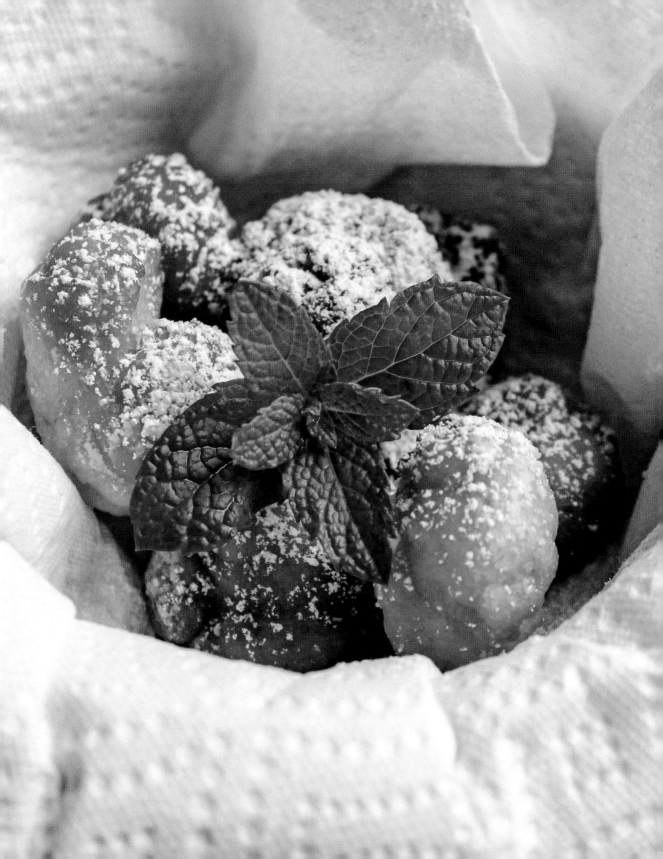

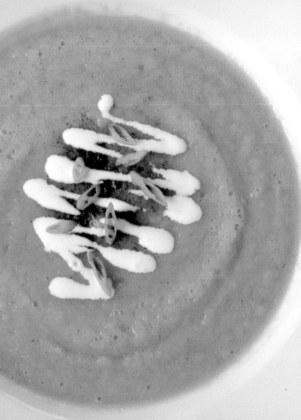

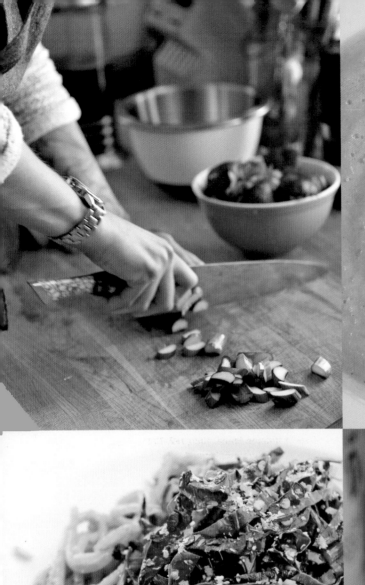

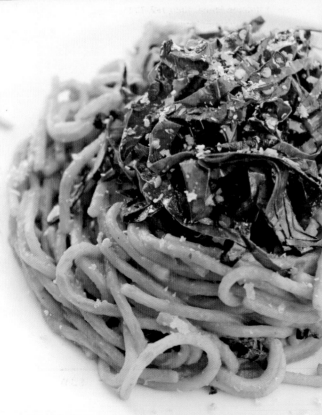

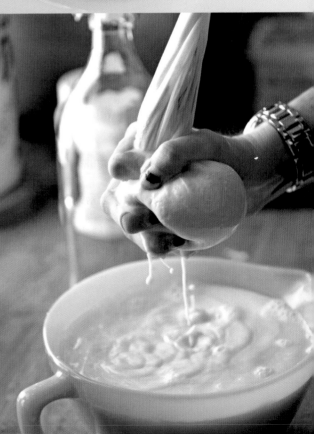

INDEX

Page numbers in *italics* indicate photographs.

A

B

bacon, 6
   B.A.L.T. Sandwich, 98, *99*
   Chive Bacon Mashed Potato Spheres, *70*, 71
   Maple Tempeh Bacon, 170, *171*
   Tempeh Bacon Spinach Quiche, 58, *59*
baking powder, baking soda, 5
Balsamic Garlic Portobello Chop, 124, *125*
balsamic vinegar, 8
Baltimore, Maryland, 1–2, 4, 12, 29, 104, 128, 139
Baltimore Sandwich, 98, *99*
bananas
   Hemp Banana Berry Muffins, 50, *51*
   Snickerdoodle Banana Bites, *52*, 53
   Sweet Banana Porridge, *40*, 41
basil, 6, 7, 9, 17
   Basil Pesto Aioli, 29
   Creamy Basil Tomato Spaghetti with Kale, 115
   Strawberry Basil Vinaigrette, *32*, 32
BBQ Quinoa Chipotle Chili, 86, *87*
BBQ Seitan Skewers, *142*, 143–44
beans, 7
   See also black beans; cannellini
"Beautiful Disaster, the" (Stuffed Artichoke), *138*, 139
Beets Quinoa Burger, The, 102, *103*
Beet Stems, Pickled (aka Lucy's Licorice), 158, *159*
bell peppers
   Bell Pepper Kale Salad, *80*, 92, *93*
   Black Bean Jambalaya, 82, *83*
   Crabby Heart Cakes, 128, *129*
   Miss Mary Macaroni Salad, 112, *113*
   Pie Wheels, *66*, 74–75, *75*
   Southwestern Scramble, 62
Benedict, California Tofu, *42*, 43
Benson's (Grandma) Blueberry Cake, 180, *181*
berries
   Blackberry Coconut Wonton Cups, *194*, 195
   Hemp Banana Berry Muffins, 50, *51*
   See also blueberry; strawberries
Beyond Meat, 7
Biscuit, Buttermilk, 150, *151*
Biscuit Muffins, Rosemary Olive Oil, 169
black beans, 7
   Beets Quinoa Burger, The, 102, *103*

   Black Bean Jambalaya, 82, *83*
   Chipotle BBQ Quinoa Chili, 86, *87*
Blackberry Coconut Wonton Cups, *194*, 195
black pepper, 6
black tofu, organic, 7
blenders, 10, 15
Blueberry Cake, Grandma Benson's, 180, *181*
Blueberry Oatmeal Squares, 46, *47*
Bob's Red Mill, 5, 6, 7, 143
Bow Ties, Firefighter's, *120*, 121
Bragg, 6, 8
Brazier, Brendan, 4
bread, 97
   Gingerbread French Toast, *36*, 48, 49
   Grandma Mattern's Date Nut Bread, 179
   See also sandwiches
bread crumbs
   Crabby Heart Cakes, 128
   Fried Eggplant Sticks, *78*, 79
   Half-Baked Macaroni and Cheese, 13, *110*, 111
   Southern Fried Buttermilk Tofu, 145
   Stuffed Artichoke ("Beautiful Disaster, the"), *138*, 139
breakfast, 37–65
   Blueberry Oatmeal Squares, 46, *47*
   Breakfast Bruschetta, 64
   California Tofu Benedict, *42*, 43
   Classic Pancakes, 38, *39*
   Crème de la Crepes, 44
   Gingerbread French Toast, *36*, 48, 49
   Glucky Waffles, The, 45
   Hemp Banana Berry Muffins, 50, *51*
   Maple Breakfast Quinoa, 60, *61*
   Snickerdoodle Banana Bites, *52*, 53
   Southwestern Scramble, 62
   Sweet Banana Porridge, *40*, 41
   Sweet Potato Waffle Sandwich, 64, *65*
   Tempeh Bacon Spinach Quiche, 58, *59*
   Traditional Glazed Doughnuts, 55–57, *56*
   Vanilla Cream, 57
   See also vegan cooking
breast cancer awareness, 4
Broth, Vegetable, 19
Brownies, Double Trouble, *186*, 187
brown sugar, organic, 7
Bruschetta, Breakfast, 64
Brussels Sprouts, Dreamy, *152*, 153

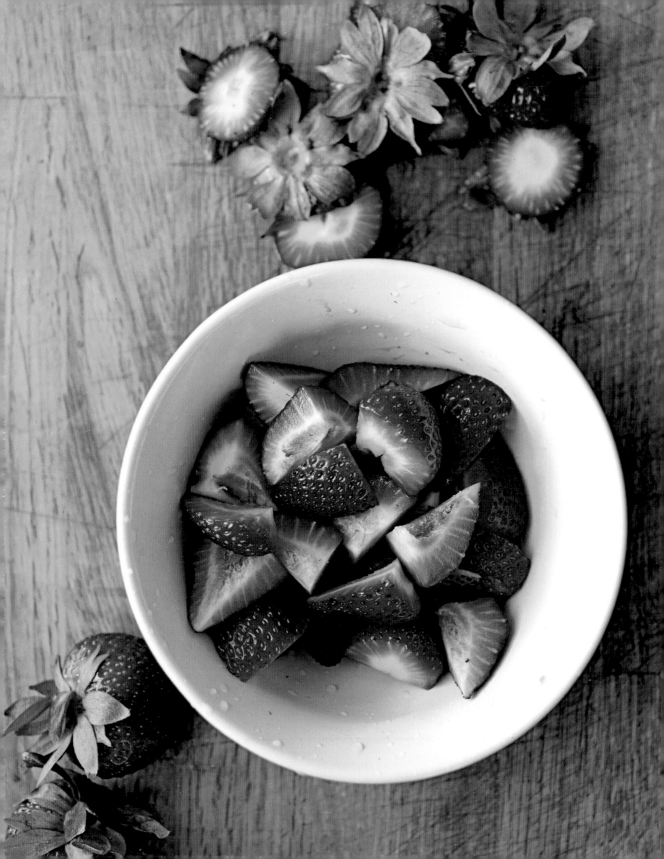